# How to Perform Isometric Exercises

A Comprehensive Guide to Building Strength, Muscle, and Endurance Without Movement - Featuring Static Contraction Training Techniques for Fitness Enthusiasts and Athletes

**Manuel Hayes**

# Table of Contents

# Introduction

**The Power of Isometric Exercises: Unleashing Your Body's Potential**

Hey there, fitness enthusiast! I know you've been searching for a way to take your strength and fitness to the next level, and I'm thrilled to tell you that you've just stumbled upon the secret weapon you've been looking for - isometric exercises!

Now, I know what you might be thinking: "Isometric exercises? Aren't those just some boring, static holds that don't really do much?" Trust me, I used to think the same thing. But after diving deep into the science behind these incredible exercises and experiencing their transformative power firsthand, I can confidently say that isometric exercises are the real deal.

Imagine being able to build strength, muscle, and endurance without even moving a muscle. Sounds too good to be true, right? But that's precisely what isometric exercises allow you to do. By harnessing the power of static contraction training, you can unlock your body's hidden potential and achieve results you never thought possible.

**My Journey: From Skeptic to Isometric Advocate**

I'll be honest with you - I wasn't always a believer in isometric exercises. As a fitness enthusiast and athlete, I was always on the lookout for the latest and greatest training methods. I tried everything from high-intensity interval training to weightlifting, but I always felt like something was missing.

That all changed when I discovered isometric exercises. At first, I was skeptical. How could simply holding a position lead to any real gains? But as I began incorporating isometric exercises into my training routine, I quickly realized just how powerful they could be.

Within weeks, I noticed improvements in my strength, stability, and overall performance. I was hooked! I began researching the science behind isometric exercises and was blown away by the evidence supporting their effectiveness. From that moment on, I became a passionate advocate for isometric training, and I've made it my mission to share this incredible method with as many people as possible.

**What You'll Gain from This Book**
If you're ready to take your fitness to new heights and experience the transformative power of isometric exercises for yourself, then this book is for you. Inside, you'll discover:

- The science behind isometric exercises and how they work to build strength, muscle, and endurance
- Step-by-step guides to the most effective isometric exercises for every muscle group
- Progressions and variations to keep your workouts challenging and engaging
- Complete isometric exercise programs for beginners, intermediates, and advanced fitness enthusiasts
- Strategies for integrating isometric exercises into your lifestyle, no matter how busy you are
- Nutritional advice and recovery tips to optimize your results and avoid burnout

- Inspiring success stories and case studies from real people who have transformed their bodies and lives with isometric exercises

Whether you're a seasoned athlete looking to take your performance to the next level, or a fitness newbie searching for a simple and effective way to get in shape, this book has something for you. So what are you waiting for? Dive in, and let's unleash your body's potential together!

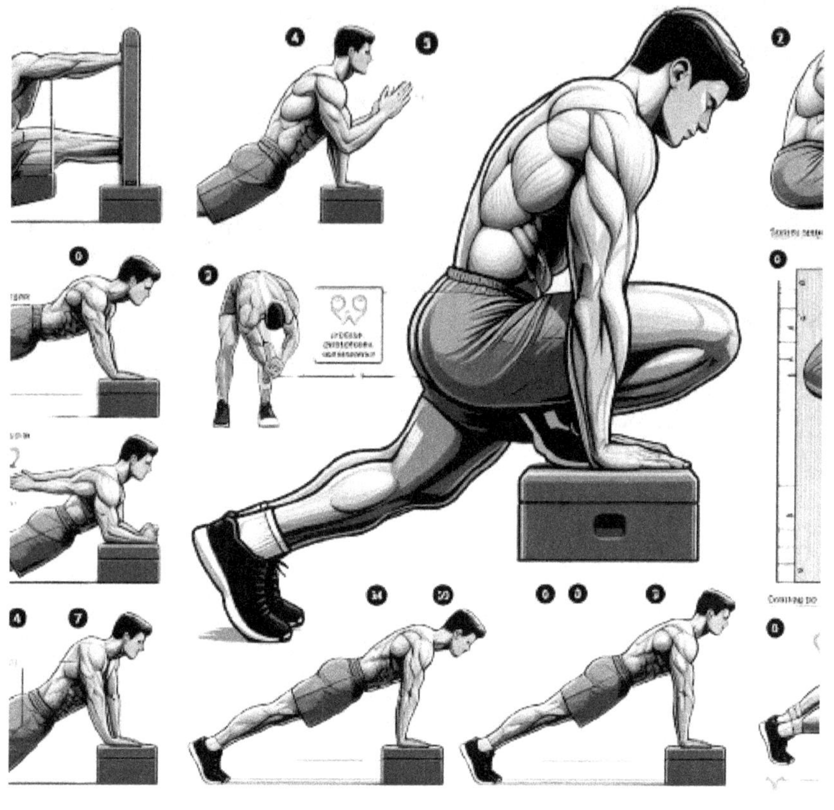

Alright, let's dive into the nitty-gritty of isometric exercises! Picture this: you're in a position where your muscles are engaged, but you're not actually moving. You're contracting your muscles without any visible joint movement. That, my friend, is the essence of an isometric exercise!

Isometric exercises, also known as static strength training, involve muscular actions in which the length of the muscle remains constant, and the joints don't move. In other words, you're putting your muscles to work without any dynamic movement. This is in contrast to concentric and eccentric muscle contractions, where the muscle length changes during the exercise.

But why would anyone want to do exercises without moving? Great question! Isometric exercises offer a unique set of benefits that traditional dynamic exercises can't always provide. Here's a breakdown of what makes isometric exercises so special:

### 1. Maximum Muscle Fiber Recruitment

When you perform an isometric exercise, you're able to recruit a high number of muscle fibers continuously. This is because you're not limited by the strength curve of a particular movement. In dynamic exercises, there are certain points where the muscle is stronger or weaker due to leverage factors. But with isometric exercises, you can maintain maximum muscle fiber recruitment throughout the entire duration of the exercise.

## 2. Increased Time Under Tension

Isometric exercises allow you to maintain muscle tension for an extended period. This increased time under tension is a key factor in building strength and muscle. By keeping your muscles engaged for longer durations, you're forcing them to adapt and grow stronger.

## 3. Joint Angle Specificity

One of the unique aspects of isometric exercises is their joint angle specificity. When you perform an isometric exercise at a particular joint angle, you're developing strength specifically at that angle. This can be particularly beneficial for athletes who need to develop strength in specific positions related to their sport.

## 4. Reduced Joint Stress

Since there's no movement during isometric exercises, there's less stress placed on the joints compared to dynamic exercises. This can be particularly beneficial for individuals with joint issues or those recovering from an injury. Isometric exercises allow you to strengthen the muscles around a joint without putting it through a full range of motion.

## 5. Versatility and Convenience

Isometric exercises can be performed anywhere, at any time, without the need for any special equipment. You can do them at home, at work, or even while traveling.

They're a convenient way to sneak in some extra strength training throughout the day.

Now that you have a better understanding of what isometric exercises are and what makes them unique, let's take a look at some common examples:

Plank: This classic core exercise involves holding your body in a straight line from head to toe, engaging your abs, back, and glutes.

- Wall Sit: With your back against a wall, lower yourself into a seated position with your knees bent at a 90-degree angle. Hold this position to target your quads, glutes, and core.

- Push-Up Hold: Get into a push-up position and lower yourself halfway down. Hold this position, maintaining tension in your chest, shoulders, and triceps.

- Glute Bridge Hold: Lie on your back with your knees bent and feet flat on the floor. Raise your hips off the ground and hold, squeezing your glutes and engaging your core.

These are just a few examples of the many isometric exercises you can incorporate into your training routine. As you progress through this book, you'll discover a wide variety of isometric exercises targeting different muscle groups and catering to various fitness levels.

Get ready to experience the power of isometric exercises firsthand! In the next chapter, we'll dive into the science behind static contraction training and explore the numerous benefits it can offer for your strength, muscle development, and overall fitness. Let's do this!

Now that you've got a solid understanding of what isometric exercises are, let's take a closer look at the science behind static contraction training. Buckle up, because we're about to geek out on some fascinating muscle physiology!

Static contraction training, as we mentioned earlier, involves holding a muscle in a contracted position without any joint movement. This type of training has some unique physiological effects on the body that contribute to its effectiveness in building strength and muscle. Let's break it down:

## 1. Muscle Fiber Recruitment

When you perform a static contraction, you're able to recruit a high number of muscle fibers right from the start. This is because you're not limited by the strength curve of a particular movement, as you are with dynamic exercises. In dynamic exercises, the number of muscle fibers recruited varies throughout the range of motion due to changes in leverage.

But with static contractions, you can recruit a maximal number of muscle fibers and maintain that recruitment throughout the duration of the exercise. This is particularly true for high-intensity isometric exercises, where you're contracting the muscle with maximum effort.

## 2. Increased Muscle Tension

One of the key factors in building strength and muscle is mechanical tension. Mechanical tension refers to the amount of force that a muscle fiber generates when it contracts. The greater the tension, the greater the stimulus for the muscle to adapt and grow stronger.

Static contraction training allows you to maintain high levels of muscle tension for an extended period. This increased time under tension is a potent stimulus for strength and muscle development. By keeping the muscle fibers contracted without any movement, you're subjecting them to a high level of mechanical tension that triggers adaptations.

## 3. Neural Adaptations

In addition to mechanical tension, static contraction training also elicits neural adaptations that contribute to strength gains. When you perform a maximal isometric contraction, you're activating a high number of motor units, which are the functional units of the nervous system that control muscle fibers.

By repeatedly activating these motor units during static contractions, you're improving your body's ability to recruit muscle fibers efficiently. This enhanced neural drive can lead to increased strength and improved coordination between the nervous system and the muscles.

## 4. Metabolic Stress

Another factor that contributes to muscle growth is metabolic stress. Metabolic stress refers to the accumulation of metabolites, such as lactate, hydrogen ions, and inorganic phosphate, within the muscle during exercise.

During static contraction training, the sustained muscle contraction can lead to a buildup of these metabolites. This creates a hypoxic environment within the muscle, meaning there's a lack of oxygen available to the muscle fibers. This metabolic stress has been shown to stimulate the release of growth factors and hormones that promote muscle growth, such as growth hormone and insulin-like growth factor-1 (IGF-1).

## 5. Reduced Joint Stress

One of the unique benefits of static contraction training is the reduced stress it places on the joints compared to dynamic exercises. During dynamic exercises, the joints are subjected to shear forces and compressive loads as they move through a range of motion.

But with static contractions, there's no joint movement, which means there's minimal shear force and compressive load on the joints. This can be particularly beneficial for individuals with joint issues or those recovering from an injury. Static contraction training allows you to strengthen the muscles around a joint without subjecting it to the same level of stress as dynamic exercises.

Now, I know that was a lot of science to digest, but understanding the physiological mechanisms behind static contraction training can help you appreciate its effectiveness and potential applications.

In the next section, we'll explore the numerous benefits of isometric exercises in more detail, including how they can help you build strength, muscle, endurance, and more. Get ready to be amazed by the transformative power of static contraction training!

## Building Strength and Muscle

Alright, it's time to dive into one of the most exciting benefits of isometric exercises: building strength and muscle! If you're looking to get stronger, sculpt your physique, and improve your overall fitness, then isometric exercises are an incredibly effective tool to have in your arsenal.

Let's take a closer look at how isometric exercises can help you build strength and muscle:

### 1. Maximum Muscle Fiber Recruitment

One of the key factors in building strength and muscle is recruiting as many muscle fibers as possible during an exercise. The more muscle fibers you can activate, the greater the stimulus for those fibers to adapt and grow stronger.

Isometric exercises are particularly effective at recruiting a high number of muscle fibers, especially when performed at a high intensity. When you perform a maximal isometric contraction, you're able to activate a greater proportion of your muscle fibers compared to dynamic exercises, where the number of fibers recruited varies throughout the range of motion.

This maximum muscle fiber recruitment during isometric exercises means you're providing a potent stimulus for strength and muscle development. By regularly engaging a high number of muscle fibers, you're forcing your body to adapt and grow stronger over time.

## 2. Increased Time Under Tension

Another crucial factor in building strength and muscle is the amount of time your muscles are under tension during an exercise. The longer your muscles are subjected to tension, the greater the stimulus for them to adapt and grow.

Isometric exercises allow you to maintain muscle tension for an extended period, often longer than you could with dynamic exercises. By holding a muscle in a contracted position, you're keeping those muscle fibers under constant tension, which is a powerful stimulus for strength and muscle growth.

This increased time under tension during isometric exercises leads to greater muscle protein synthesis, which is the process by which your body builds new muscle tissue. By subjecting your muscles to longer periods of tension, you're triggering the physiological processes that lead to muscle growth and development.

## 3. Overcoming Sticking Points

In dynamic exercises, there are often specific points in the range of motion where you're weaker and more likely to fail. These points, known as sticking points, can limit your overall strength and muscle development.

Isometric exercises allow you to target these sticking points specifically and develop strength in those particular positions. By performing isometric contractions at your sticking points, you can improve your strength and stability in those specific joint angles.

For example, if you tend to struggle with the bottom portion of a squat, performing isometric holds in that bottom position can help you develop the strength and control needed to overcome that sticking point. This can translate to improved performance in your dynamic squats and overall lower body strength.

## 4. Muscle Hypertrophy

In addition to strength development, isometric exercises can also contribute to muscle hypertrophy, which is the increase in muscle size. While dynamic exercises are typically emphasized for hypertrophy, isometric exercises can play a valuable role as well.

The high levels of muscle tension and increased time under tension during isometric exercises can stimulate muscle protein synthesis and lead to muscle growth. Additionally, the metabolic stress generated during isometric contractions, as we discussed in the previous section, can promote the release of growth factors and hormones that support muscle hypertrophy.

Incorporating isometric exercises alongside your dynamic training can provide a unique stimulus for muscle growth and help you achieve a well-rounded physique.

## 5. Improved Mind-Muscle Connection

One of the often-overlooked benefits of isometric exercises is their ability to improve your mind-muscle connection. The mind-muscle connection refers to your ability to consciously engage and contract a specific muscle group during an exercise.

During isometric exercises, you have the opportunity to focus intently on the muscle you're targeting and develop a greater sense of control and activation. By holding a muscle in a contracted position, you can really zone in on the sensation of that muscle working and establish a stronger neurological connection.

This improved mind-muscle connection can translate to better muscle activation and control during your dynamic exercises as well. By developing a greater sense of how to engage a specific muscle group, you can improve your form, increase the effectiveness of your exercises, and potentially reduce your risk of injury.

Building strength and muscle is a journey, and isometric exercises can be a powerful tool to help you reach your destination. By harnessing the benefits of maximum muscle fiber recruitment, increased time under tension, overcoming sticking points, muscle hypertrophy, and improved mind-muscle connection, you can take your strength and physique to new heights.

In the next section, we'll explore how isometric exercises can also help you develop endurance and improve your overall fitness. Get ready to discover the incredible versatility of isometric training!

# Enhancing Endurance

Now that we've explored how isometric exercises can help you build strength and muscle, let's dive into another incredible benefit: enhancing endurance! Whether you're an athlete looking to improve your performance or simply someone who wants to increase their stamina and resilience, isometric exercises can be a game-changer.

Endurance refers to your body's ability to sustain physical activity for an extended period. It's the foundation of many athletic pursuits and is crucial for maintaining overall health and wellness. Isometric exercises can play a significant role in developing and enhancing your endurance in several ways.

Let's take a closer look at how isometric exercises can boost your endurance:

## 1. Improving Muscular Endurance

Muscular endurance refers to a muscle's ability to sustain repeated contractions or maintain a single contraction for an extended period. It's essential for activities that require prolonged muscle activation, such as running, cycling, or swimming.

Isometric exercises are particularly effective at improving muscular endurance because they involve sustaining a muscle contraction for a significant duration. By holding a muscle in a contracted position, you're challenging it to maintain that tension without rest, which can lead to adaptations in muscular endurance.

For example, performing isometric holds like planks, wall sits, or glute bridges can help improve the endurance of your core, legs, and glutes, respectively. By regularly incorporating these exercises into your training routine, you can develop the ability to sustain muscle contractions for longer periods, translating to improved performance in endurance-based activities.

## 2. Enhancing Cardiovascular Endurance

While isometric exercises primarily target muscular endurance, they can also have a positive impact on your cardiovascular endurance. Cardiovascular endurance refers to your heart, lungs, and blood vessels' ability to supply oxygen to your muscles during sustained physical activity.

During isometric exercises, your muscles are in a state of constant tension, which places a demand on your cardiovascular system to deliver oxygen and nutrients to those working muscles. As you hold an isometric contraction, your heart rate increases, and your breathing becomes more challenging, similar to what you might experience during aerobic exercise.

Over time, regularly engaging in isometric exercises can lead to adaptations in your cardiovascular system. Your heart becomes more efficient at pumping blood, your blood vessels become more elastic and responsive, and your body becomes better at utilizing oxygen. These adaptations can translate to improved cardiovascular endurance, allowing you to sustain physical activity for longer periods without fatigue.

## 3. Developing Mental Endurance

Endurance isn't just about physical adaptations; it also has a significant mental component. Mental endurance refers to your ability to push through discomfort, maintain focus, and stay motivated during challenging physical activities.

Isometric exercises can be a powerful tool for developing mental endurance. When you're holding an isometric contraction, especially for an extended period, you're forced to confront and push through the discomfort and fatigue that inevitably arise. This requires mental toughness and the ability to stay focused on the task at hand.

By regularly engaging in isometric exercises and progressively increasing the duration of your holds, you can develop a greater tolerance for discomfort and improve your mental resilience. This mental endurance can translate to improved performance in other areas of your life, both in and out of the gym.

## 4. Enhancing Postural Endurance

Postural endurance refers to your ability to maintain proper posture and alignment during prolonged activities, such as sitting at a desk or standing for extended periods. Poor postural endurance can lead to discomfort, fatigue, and even injury over time.

Isometric exercises can be an effective way to improve your postural endurance. By targeting the muscles responsible for maintaining proper posture, such as the core, upper back, and glutes, you can develop the strength and endurance needed to sustain good alignment throughout the day.

For example, performing isometric exercises like planks, bird dogs, or glute bridges can help strengthen the muscles that support your spine and pelvis. By regularly incorporating these exercises into your routine, you can improve your ability to maintain proper posture during extended periods of sitting or standing, reducing your risk of discomfort and injury.

## 5. Complementing Dynamic Training

While isometric exercises can be highly effective for developing endurance on their own, they can also serve as a valuable complement to dynamic training. Incorporating isometric exercises alongside your regular endurance training can provide a unique stimulus for adaptation and help you break through plateaus.

For example, if you're a runner looking to improve your endurance, you might incorporate isometric holds like wall sits or single-leg glute bridges into your training routine. These exercises can help strengthen the muscles involved in running, improve your stability and control, and enhance your overall endurance.

Similarly, if you're engaged in a strength training program, adding isometric exercises can help you develop greater muscular endurance and improve your ability to maintain proper form and tension throughout your dynamic exercises.

Enhancing endurance is a multifaceted pursuit, and isometric exercises can be a valuable tool in your arsenal. By improving muscular endurance, cardiovascular endurance, mental endurance, postural endurance, and complementing your dynamic training, isometric exercises can help you become a more resilient, capable, and well-rounded athlete.

In the next section, we'll explore the convenience and versatility of isometric exercises, and how you can incorporate them into your training routine no matter your fitness level or goals. Get ready to discover the power of isometric training in your own life!

# Improving Joint Stability

When it comes to building a strong, resilient, and injury-resistant body, joint stability is a crucial piece of the puzzle. Your joints are the connection points between your bones, allowing for movement and providing support for your body. Isometric exercises can play a significant role in improving joint stability, helping you move more efficiently, reduce your risk of injury, and enhance your overall quality of life.

Let's take a closer look at how isometric exercises can improve joint stability:

## 1. Strengthening the Muscles Around the Joint

One of the primary ways isometric exercises improve joint stability is by strengthening the muscles that surround and support the joint. When the muscles around a joint are strong and well-developed, they provide greater support and stability to the joint itself.

For example, consider the knee joint. The knee is supported by several key muscle groups, including the quadriceps, hamstrings, and calves. By performing isometric exercises like wall sits or single-leg glute bridges, you can target and strengthen these muscle groups, providing greater stability to the knee joint.

Similarly, isometric exercises can help strengthen the muscles around other joints, such as the shoulders, hips, and ankles. By developing strong, supportive muscles, you can reduce the stress placed on the joints themselves and improve their overall stability.

## 2. Enhancing Neuromuscular Control

Joint stability isn't just about strength; it's also about control. Neuromuscular control refers to your body's ability to coordinate and control the muscles around a joint, allowing for precise, stable movement.

Isometric exercises can be highly effective at improving neuromuscular control. When you perform an isometric contraction, you're challenging your body to maintain a specific position against resistance. This requires a high degree of muscle activation and control, as you work to stabilize the joint and maintain proper alignment.

Over time, regularly engaging in isometric exercises can lead to improvements in neuromuscular control. Your body becomes more efficient at recruiting the appropriate muscles, coordinating their activation, and maintaining stability throughout the movement. This enhanced control can translate to improved joint stability during dynamic activities as well.

## 3. Improving Proprioception

Proprioception refers to your body's ability to sense its position and movement in space. It's the feedback loop between your muscles, joints, and nervous system that allows you to maintain balance, coordinate movement, and adjust to changes in your environment.

Isometric exercises can be a powerful tool for improving proprioception, particularly around the joints. When you perform an isometric contraction, you're providing your body with a specific stimulus – a static, controlled position that requires muscle activation and joint stability.

As you hold this position, your body is constantly receiving feedback from your muscles and joints about their position and the forces acting upon them. This feedback helps refine your proprioception, making you more aware of your body's position and movement in space.

Over time, regular isometric training can lead to improvements in proprioception, allowing you to more effectively sense and control your joints during movement. This enhanced proprioception can contribute to greater joint stability and a reduced risk of injury.

## 4. Reducing Joint Stress

One of the unique benefits of isometric exercises is their ability to strengthen the muscles around a joint without placing excessive stress on the joint itself. This is particularly valuable for individuals with joint issues, such as arthritis or previous injuries.

During dynamic exercises, the joints are subjected to shear forces and compressive loads as they move through a range of motion. While these forces are a normal part of movement, they can be problematic for individuals with compromised joint health.

Isometric exercises, on the other hand, allow you to strengthen the muscles around a joint without subjecting it to the same level of stress. By holding a static position, you can target and strengthen the supporting muscles without placing undue strain on the joint itself.

This reduced joint stress can be especially beneficial for individuals who are recovering from an injury or dealing with chronic joint pain. Isometric exercises provide a safe, controlled way to build strength and stability around the affected joint, without exacerbating existing issues.

## 5. Enhancing Functional Movement

Ultimately, the goal of improving joint stability is to enhance your ability to perform functional movements safely and efficiently. Functional movements are the movements you perform in daily life, such as walking, squatting, reaching, and lifting.

Isometric exercises can play a valuable role in improving functional movement by developing the strength, control, and stability needed to perform these movements with proper form and technique. By targeting the specific muscles and joint angles involved in functional movements, you can build a foundation of stability that translates to improved performance in everyday life.

For example, performing isometric holds in a deep squat position can help develop the strength and stability needed to perform squatting movements safely and efficiently. Similarly, isometric exercises targeting the shoulder joint can improve your ability to reach and lift objects overhead without compromising joint health.

Improving joint stability is a critical component of overall health and wellness. By strengthening the muscles around the joints, enhancing neuromuscular control, improving proprioception, reducing joint stress, and enhancing functional movement, isometric exercises can play a powerful role in building a strong, resilient, and injury-resistant body.

In the next section, we'll explore the convenience and versatility of isometric exercises, and how you can easily incorporate them into your daily routine to reap the benefits of improved joint stability and overall health. Get ready to discover the power of isometric training in supporting your joints and enhancing your quality of life!

# Convenience and Versatility

One of the most appealing aspects of isometric exercises is their convenience and versatility. Unlike many other forms of exercise that require specialized equipment, dedicated facilities, or significant time commitments, isometric exercises can be performed almost anywhere, anytime, with minimal equipment. This makes them an incredibly accessible and practical addition to any fitness routine.

Let's dive into the convenience and versatility of isometric exercises in more detail:

## 1. Minimal Equipment Required

Isometric exercises are unique in that they require little to no equipment to perform effectively. While some exercises may benefit from the use of simple tools like resistance bands or stability balls, the vast majority of isometric exercises can be performed using only your body weight and a stable surface.

This means you can engage in isometric training at home, at the office, in a hotel room, or even outdoors. You don't need to invest in expensive gym memberships, bulky weightlifting equipment, or specialized machines. With just your body and a few square feet of space, you can engage in a full-body isometric workout that challenges your strength, stability, and endurance.

## 2. Time Efficiency

In today's fast-paced world, time is a precious commodity. Many people struggle to find the time to dedicate to lengthy workouts or complex training routines.

Isometric exercises offer a solution to this problem by providing a time-efficient way to build strength, stability, and endurance.

Because isometric exercises involve holding a static position, they can be performed in short bursts throughout the day. A single isometric hold may only take 30 seconds to a few minutes, making it easy to incorporate into even the busiest of schedules.

For example, you could perform a set of plank holds during a work break, do a wall sit while waiting for your coffee to brew, or engage in a glute bridge hold while watching television in the evening. By breaking your isometric training into small, manageable chunks, you can accumulate significant benefits over time without dedicating large blocks of time to your workouts.

### 3. Adaptability to Fitness Levels

Another aspect of the versatility of isometric exercises is their adaptability to different fitness levels. Whether you're a beginner just starting your fitness journey or an advanced athlete looking to take your training to the next level, isometric exercises can be modified to meet your needs.

For beginners, isometric exercises can be performed with shorter hold times and modified positions to accommodate current strength and stability levels. As you progress, you can gradually increase the duration of your holds, add complexity to the exercises, or incorporate additional resistance to continue challenging your body.

Advanced exercisers can use isometric exercises to target specific muscle groups, work on weak points in their strength or stability, or push their endurance to new limits. By adjusting variables like hold time, joint angle, and resistance, you can create an isometric training program that is tailored to your specific goals and needs.

## 4. Flexibility in Training Style

Isometric exercises also offer flexibility in terms of training style. They can be easily incorporated into a variety of training approaches, from traditional strength training routines to more holistic practices like yoga and Pilates.

For example, you could use isometric holds as part of a circuit training routine, moving from one exercise to the next with minimal rest to keep your heart rate elevated and challenge your endurance. Alternatively, you could incorporate isometric exercises into a yoga practice, using holds like chair pose or warrior III to build strength and stability in key yoga positions.

Isometric exercises can also be used as a standalone training method, focusing solely on static holds to develop strength, stability, and endurance. This approach can be particularly valuable for individuals who are recovering from an injury, have limited mobility, or simply prefer a more low-impact training style.

## 5. Convenience for Travel and On-the-Go Training

Finally, the convenience and versatility of isometric exercises make them an ideal choice for travel and on-the-go training.

Whether you're a frequent business traveler, a busy parent, or simply someone who enjoys being active outdoors, isometric exercises can help you maintain your fitness routine no matter where you are.

Because isometric exercises require minimal space and equipment, they can be easily performed in a hotel room, a park, or even on a beach. You can use furniture, walls, or even trees as support for your isometric holds, making the most of your surroundings to get in a challenging workout.

## Assessing Your Current Fitness Level

Before diving into any new exercise routine, it's essential to assess your current fitness level. This assessment serves as a starting point, helping you set realistic goals, create a safe and effective training plan, and track your progress over time. When it comes to isometric exercises, assessing your fitness level involves evaluating your strength, stability, and endurance in key areas of the body.

Let's take a closer look at how to assess your current fitness level for isometric exercises:

### 1. Evaluating Overall Strength

Strength is a fundamental component of any fitness routine, and isometric exercises are no exception. To assess your overall strength, you can perform a series of basic isometric holds and note how long you can maintain each position with proper form.

Some key isometric exercises to assess strength include:

- Plank hold: This exercise targets your core, shoulders, and back. Start in a push-up position, with your forearms on the ground and your elbows directly under your shoulders. Hold this position, keeping your body in a straight line from head to heels.

- Wall sit: This exercise targets your quadriceps, hamstrings, and glutes. Stand with your back against a wall, then slide down until your thighs are parallel to the ground. Hold this position, keeping your knees at a 90-degree angle.

- Glute bridge hold: This exercise targets your glutes and hamstrings. Lie on your back with your knees bent and your feet flat on the ground. Lift your hips off the ground until your body forms a straight line from your knees to your shoulders. Hold this position, squeezing your glutes and engaging your core.

For each of these exercises, aim to hold the position for as long as you can with proper form. Record your hold times to establish a baseline for your current strength level.

**2. Assessing Joint Stability**

Joint stability is another key factor to consider when assessing your fitness level for isometric exercises. Stable joints are essential for performing isometric holds safely and effectively, as they help prevent injury and ensure proper alignment throughout the exercise.

To assess your joint stability, you can perform a series of single-leg isometric holds and note any wobbling, shaking, or loss of balance. Some exercises to assess joint stability include:

- Wall sit: This exercise targets your quadriceps, hamstrings, and glutes. Stand with your back against a wall, then slide down until your thighs are parallel to the ground. Hold this position, keeping your knees at a 90-degree angle.

- Glute bridge hold: This exercise targets your glutes and hamstrings. Lie on your back with your knees bent and your feet flat on the ground. Lift your hips off the ground until your body forms a straight line from your knees to your shoulders. Hold this position, squeezing your glutes and engaging your core.

For each of these exercises, aim to hold the position for as long as you can with proper form. Record your hold times to establish a baseline for your current strength level.

## 2. Assessing Joint Stability

Joint stability is another key factor to consider when assessing your fitness level for isometric exercises. Stable joints are essential for performing isometric holds safely and effectively, as they help prevent injury and ensure proper alignment throughout the exercise.

To assess your joint stability, you can perform a series of single-leg isometric holds and note any wobbling, shaking, or loss of balance. Some exercises to assess joint stability include:

- Single-leg glute bridge hold: This exercise targets your glutes, hamstrings, and hip stabilizers. Lie on your back with one foot flat on the ground and the other leg extended straight up toward the ceiling. Lift your hips off the ground, holding the position while maintaining stability in your raised leg.

- Single-leg wall sit: This exercise targets your quadriceps, hamstrings, and knee stabilizers. Stand with your back against a wall, then slide down until your thighs are parallel to the ground. Lift one foot off the ground, holding the position while maintaining stability in your supporting leg.

- Single-leg balance hold: This exercise targets your ankle and hip stabilizers. Stand on one leg, keeping your raised foot off the ground and your standing knee slightly bent. Hold this position, focusing on maintaining balance and stability.

For each of these exercises, aim to hold the position for as long as you can with proper form and minimal wobbling or shaking. Note any differences in stability between your right and left sides, as this can help you identify areas that may need extra attention in your isometric training.

### 3. Evaluating Muscular Endurance

Muscular endurance refers to your muscles' ability to sustain repeated contractions or hold a single contraction for an extended period. Assessing your muscular endurance can help you determine how long you can safely and effectively perform isometric holds in your training routine.

To assess your muscular endurance, you can perform a series of isometric holds for time and note how long you can maintain each position with proper form. Some exercises to assess muscular endurance include:

- Forearm plank hold: This exercise targets your core, shoulders, and back. Start in a plank position, with your forearms on the ground and your elbows directly under your shoulders. Hold this position, keeping your body in a straight line from head to heels, for as long as you can maintain proper form.

- Wall sit hold: This exercise targets your quadriceps, hamstrings, and glutes. Stand with your back against a wall, then slide down until your thighs are parallel to the ground. Hold this position, keeping your knees at a 90-degree angle, for as long as you can maintain proper form.

- Dead hang hold: This exercise targets your grip strength, shoulders, and back. Hang from a pull-up bar with your arms fully extended and your palms facing away from you. Hold this position, engaging your shoulder blades and core, for as long as you can maintain proper form.

For each of these exercises, aim to hold the position for as long as possible without sacrificing form. Record your hold times to establish a baseline for your current muscular endurance.

## 4. Setting Realistic Goals

Once you've assessed your current fitness level in terms of strength, stability, and endurance, you can use this information to set realistic goals for your isometric training. Setting achievable goals can help you stay motivated, track your progress, and adjust your training plan as needed.

Some examples of realistic goals for isometric training might include:

- Increasing your plank hold time by 30 seconds over the course of a month
- Improving your single-leg balance hold time by 10 seconds on each side
- Maintaining proper form in a wall sit hold for an additional 15 seconds

When setting goals, be sure to consider your current fitness level, any limitations or injuries, and the amount of time you can realistically dedicate to your isometric training. Aim to set goals that are specific, measurable, achievable, relevant, and time-bound (SMART) to help ensure success.

## 5. Tracking Your Progress

As you progress through your isometric training, it's important to regularly reassess your fitness level and track your progress toward your goals. This can help you stay motivated, identify areas for improvement, and adjust your training plan as needed.

Some strategies for tracking your progress with isometric exercises include:

- Recording your hold times for each exercise in a training log or journal
- Taking progress photos or videos to visually document changes in your strength, stability, and form
- Assessing your fitness level every 4-6 weeks to measure improvements in strength, stability, and endurance
- Celebrating your achievements and milestones along the way

Remember, progress with isometric training may be gradual, but consistent effort and dedication can lead to significant improvements over time. By regularly assessing your fitness level and tracking your progress, you can stay motivated and make steady gains in your strength, stability, and endurance.

Assessing your current fitness level is a crucial first step in getting started with isometric exercises. By evaluating your strength, stability, and endurance, setting realistic goals, and tracking your progress, you can create a safe, effective, and achievable isometric training plan.

In the next section, we'll explore how to create your own isometric exercise space, including the essential equipment and accessories you may need to get started. Get ready to set yourself up for success as you embark on your isometric training journey!

Before diving into any new exercise routine, it's essential to assess your current fitness level. This assessment serves as a starting point, helping you set realistic goals, create a safe and effective training plan, and track your progress over time. When it comes to isometric exercises, assessing your fitness level involves evaluating your strength, stability, and endurance in key areas of the body.

Let's take a closer look at how to assess your current fitness level for isometric exercises:

### 1. Evaluating Overall Strength

Strength is a fundamental component of any fitness routine, and isometric exercises are no exception. To assess your overall strength, you can perform a series of basic isometric holds and note how long you can maintain each position with proper form.

Some key isometric exercises to assess strength include:

- Plank hold: This exercise targets your core, shoulders, and back. Start in a push-up position, with your forearms on the ground and your elbows directly under your shoulders. Hold this position, keeping your body in a straight line from head to heels.

- Wall sit: This exercise targets your quadriceps, hamstrings, and glutes. Stand with your back against a wall, then slide down until your thighs are parallel to the ground. Hold this position, keeping your knees at a 90-degree angle.

- Glute bridge hold: This exercise targets your glutes and hamstrings. Lie on your back with your knees bent and your feet flat on the ground. Lift your hips off the ground until your body forms a straight line from your knees to your shoulders. Hold this position, squeezing your glutes and engaging your core.

For each of these exercises, aim to hold the position for as long as you can with proper form. Record your hold times to establish a baseline for your current strength level.

## 2. Assessing Joint Stability

Joint stability is another key factor to consider when assessing your fitness level for isometric exercises. Stable joints are essential for performing isometric holds safely and effectively, as they help prevent injury and ensure proper alignment throughout the exercise.

To assess your joint stability, you can perform a series of single-leg isometric holds and note any wobbling, shaking, or loss of balance. Some exercises to assess joint stability include:

- Single-leg glute bridge hold: This exercise targets your glutes, hamstrings, and hip stabilizers. Lie on your back with one foot flat on the ground and the other leg extended straight up toward the ceiling. Lift your hips off the ground, holding the position while maintaining stability in your raised leg.

- Single-leg wall sit: This exercise targets your quadriceps, hamstrings, and knee stabilizers. Stand with your back against a wall, then slide down until your thighs are parallel to the ground. Lift one foot off the ground, holding the position while maintaining stability in your supporting leg.

- Single-leg balance hold: This exercise targets your ankle and hip stabilizers. Stand on one leg, keeping your raised foot off the ground and your standing knee slightly bent. Hold this position, focusing on maintaining balance and stability.

For each of these exercises, aim to hold the position for as long as you can with proper form and minimal wobbling or shaking. Note any differences in stability between your right and left sides, as this can help you identify areas that may need extra attention in your isometric training.

### 3. Evaluating Muscular Endurance

Muscular endurance refers to your muscles' ability to sustain repeated contractions or hold a single contraction for an extended period. Assessing your muscular endurance can help you determine how long you can safely and effectively perform isometric holds in your training routine.

To assess your muscular endurance, you can perform a series of isometric holds for time and note how long you can maintain each position with proper form. Some exercises to assess muscular endurance include:

- Forearm plank hold: This exercise targets your core, shoulders, and back. Start in a plank position, with your forearms on the ground and your elbows directly under your shoulders. Hold this position, keeping your body in a straight line from head to heels, for as long as you can maintain proper form.

- Wall sit hold: This exercise targets your quadriceps, hamstrings, and glutes. Stand with your back against a wall, then slide down until your thighs are parallel to the ground. Hold this position, keeping your knees at a 90-degree angle, for as long as you can maintain proper form.

- Dead hang hold: This exercise targets your grip strength, shoulders, and back. Hang from a pull-up bar with your arms fully extended and your palms facing away from you. Hold this position, engaging your shoulder blades and core, for as long as you can maintain proper form.

For each of these exercises, aim to hold the position for as long as possible without sacrificing form. Record your hold times to establish a baseline for your current muscular endurance.

## 4. Setting Realistic Goals

Once you've assessed your current fitness level in terms of strength, stability, and endurance, you can use this information to set realistic goals for your isometric training. Setting achievable goals can help you stay motivated, track your progress, and adjust your training plan as needed.

Some examples of realistic goals for isometric training might include:

- Increasing your plank hold time by 30 seconds over the course of a month
- Improving your single-leg balance hold time by 10 seconds on each side
- Maintaining proper form in a wall sit hold for an additional 15 seconds

When setting goals, be sure to consider your current fitness level, any limitations or injuries, and the amount of time you can realistically dedicate to your isometric training. Aim to set goals that are specific, measurable, achievable, relevant, and time-bound (SMART) to help ensure success.

## 5. Tracking Your Progress

As you progress through your isometric training, it's important to regularly reassess your fitness level and track your progress toward your goals. This can help you stay motivated, identify areas for improvement, and adjust your training plan as needed.

Some strategies for tracking your progress with isometric exercises include:

- Recording your hold times for each exercise in a training log or journal
- Taking progress photos or videos to visually document changes in your strength, stability, and form

- Assessing your fitness level every 4-6 weeks to measure improvements in strength, stability, and endurance
- Celebrating your achievements and milestones along the way

Remember, progress with isometric training may be gradual, but consistent effort and dedication can lead to significant improvements over time. By regularly assessing your fitness level and tracking your progress, you can stay motivated and make steady gains in your strength, stability, and endurance.

Assessing your current fitness level is a crucial first step in getting started with isometric exercises. By evaluating your strength, stability, and endurance, setting realistic goals, and tracking your progress, you can create a safe, effective, and achievable isometric training plan.

In the next section, we'll explore how to create your own isometric exercise space, including the essential equipment and accessories you may need to get started. Get ready to set yourself up for success as you embark on your isometric training journey!

One of the great advantages of isometric exercises is that they can be performed almost anywhere, with minimal equipment. However, creating a dedicated space for your isometric training can help you stay focused, motivated, and consistent with your workouts. By setting up a comfortable, functional, and inviting exercise area, you'll be more likely to stick to your training plan and achieve your fitness goals.

Let's explore some key considerations for creating your ideal isometric exercise space:

### 1. Choosing a Location

The first step in creating your isometric exercise space is choosing a suitable location. Look for an area in your home, office, or outdoor space that offers enough room to move freely and hold various isometric positions comfortably.

Some factors to consider when choosing a location include:

- Space: Ensure you have enough floor space to lie down, stretch, and perform isometric holds without feeling cramped or restricted.
- Privacy: If possible, choose a location that offers some privacy, so you can focus on your exercises without distractions or interruptions.
- Lighting: Aim for a well-lit space that allows you to see your form clearly and maintain proper alignment throughout your isometric holds.
- Ventilation: Select a location with good ventilation to help you stay cool and comfortable during your workouts.

- Accessibility: Consider choosing a space that's easily accessible and convenient, so you're more likely to use it regularly.

Some examples of suitable locations for an isometric exercise space might include a spare room, a corner of your bedroom, a section of your living room, or even a quiet spot in your backyard or local park.

## 2. Flooring and Surfaces

The type of flooring or surface you choose for your isometric exercise space can have a big impact on your comfort, safety, and performance. Ideally, you'll want a surface that's firm, stable, and provides some cushioning for your joints.

Some options for isometric exercise flooring include:

- Yoga mats: A high-quality yoga mat can provide a comfortable, non-slip surface for your isometric holds and stretches.
- Interlocking foam tiles: These tiles can be easily assembled to create a cushioned, supportive surface for your workouts.
- Carpeting: If you have a carpeted area in your home, this can provide a suitable surface for isometric exercises, as long as the carpet is not too thick or plush.
- Hardwood or laminate flooring: These surfaces can work well for isometric exercises, but you may want to use a yoga mat or other padding to provide some cushioning for your joints.

When selecting a flooring option, consider factors like durability, ease of cleaning, and the specific demands of your isometric training plan.

## 3. Essential Equipment

While isometric exercises can be performed with minimal equipment, having a few key tools on hand can help you get the most out of your workouts. Some essential equipment for your isometric exercise space might include:

- Yoga mat or other non-slip flooring
- Resistance bands: These versatile tools can be used to add resistance to your isometric holds and stretches, allowing you to progress your workouts over time.
- Stability ball: A stability ball can be used to add an element of instability to your isometric holds, challenging your core and improving your balance.
- Foam roller: A foam roller can be used for self-myofascial release and muscle recovery before and after your isometric workouts.
- Timer: A simple timer or stopwatch can help you track your hold times and rest periods during your isometric exercises.

Consider your specific fitness goals and training plan when selecting equipment for your isometric exercise space, and invest in high-quality tools that will last over time.

## 4. Storage Solutions

To keep your isometric exercise space organized and clutter-free, it's important to have some storage solutions on hand. This might include:

- A basket or bin for storing your yoga mat, resistance bands, and other small equipment
- A shelving unit or cabinet for larger items like stability balls or foam rollers
- Wall-mounted hooks or racks for hanging resistance bands, towels, or other accessories

By keeping your equipment organized and easily accessible, you'll be more likely to use your isometric exercise space regularly and stay on track with your training plan.

## 5. Creating a Motivating Atmosphere

Finally, consider adding some personal touches to your isometric exercise space to make it feel more inviting and motivating. This might include:

- Inspiring artwork or posters featuring your favorite athletes, quotes, or landscapes
- Plants or other natural elements to bring a sense of calm and tranquility to your space
- A sound system or speakers for playing your favorite workout music or guided meditation tracks
- Aromatherapy diffusers or candles to create a pleasant, relaxing scent
- A whiteboard or cork board for tracking your progress, setting goals, or posting affirmations

By creating a space that feels personalized and inspiring, you'll be more likely to look forward to your isometric workouts and stay committed to your fitness journey.

Creating your ideal isometric exercise space is all about finding a location, flooring, equipment, and atmosphere that work for you. By taking the time to set up a dedicated area for your workouts, you'll be setting yourself up for success and making it easier to stay consistent with your isometric training.

In the next section, we'll dive into the essential equipment and accessories you may want to consider adding to your isometric exercise space, and how to use them to get the most out of your workouts. Get ready to take your isometric training to the next level!

When it comes to isometric exercises, one of the great advantages is that you don't need a lot of fancy equipment to get started. However, having a few key tools on hand can help you get the most out of your workouts, stay comfortable and safe, and progress your training over time.

Let's take a closer look at some essential equipment and accessories for your isometric exercise routine:

**1. Yoga Mat or Non-Slip Flooring**
A high-quality yoga mat or non-slip flooring is arguably the most essential piece of equipment for your isometric exercise space. A good mat will provide a stable, comfortable surface for your workouts, helping you maintain proper form and alignment while also protecting your joints from hard surfaces.

When choosing a yoga mat, look for one that is:

- Thick enough to provide cushioning and support, but not so thick that it affects your balance or stability
- Made from a non-slip material that will keep you stable during your isometric holds and stretches
- Durable and easy to clean, so it will last through many workouts and stay hygienic over time

If you prefer not to use a yoga mat, you can also invest in other non-slip flooring options like interlocking foam tiles or a large, non-slip exercise mat.

## 2. Resistance Bands

Resistance bands are a versatile and portable tool that can be used to add resistance to your isometric holds and stretches. By incorporating resistance bands into your workouts, you can challenge your muscles in new ways, improve your strength and stability, and progress your training over time.

Some ways to use resistance bands in your isometric exercises include:

- Looping the band around your legs or feet during a plank hold to add resistance and engage your core and lower body muscles
- Holding the ends of the band in each hand during a wall sit to add resistance and target your quadriceps and glutes
- Anchoring the band to a sturdy object and holding the ends during a standing row hold to target your back and shoulder muscles

When choosing resistance bands, look for a set that includes multiple levels of resistance (such as light, medium, and heavy) so you can progress your workouts over time. You may also want to choose bands with comfortable handles or anchors for easy gripping and setup.

## 3. Stability Ball

A stability ball, also known as an exercise ball or Swiss ball, is another versatile tool that can be used to add an element of instability to your isometric holds. By performing exercises on a stability ball, you'll engage your core muscles and improve your balance and coordination while also targeting specific muscle groups.

Some ways to use a stability ball in your isometric exercises include:

- Performing a plank hold with your forearms resting on the ball, engaging your core and shoulder muscles to maintain balance
- Sitting on the ball during a wall sit, engaging your core and leg muscles to maintain stability and proper form
- Lying on the ball during a glute bridge hold, engaging your core and glute muscles to keep the ball stable and your body in alignment

When choosing a stability ball, look for one that is appropriately sized for your height (you should be able to sit on the ball with your feet flat on the ground and your knees at a 90-degree angle). You may also want to choose a ball with a non-slip surface for added stability during your workouts.

## 4. Foam Roller

A foam roller is a simple but effective tool for self-myofascial release and muscle recovery. By using a foam roller before and after your isometric workouts, you can help reduce muscle tension, improve flexibility, and promote blood flow to your muscles.

Some ways to use a foam roller in your isometric exercise routine include:

- Rolling out your quadriceps, hamstrings, and calves before a leg-focused isometric workout to improve flexibility and reduce the risk of injury
- Rolling out your upper back and shoulders after a plank or push-up hold to release tension and promote recovery

- Rolling out your glutes and hip muscles after a glute bridge or wall sit hold to reduce tightness and improve mobility

When choosing a foam roller, look for one that is firm enough to provide deep tissue pressure, but not so hard that it causes pain or discomfort. You may also want to choose a roller with a textured surface for added intensity and targeted muscle release.

## 5. Timer or Stopwatch

A simple timer or stopwatch is an essential accessory for tracking your hold times and rest periods during your isometric exercises. By using a timer, you can ensure that you're holding each position for the appropriate amount of time, and taking adequate rest breaks between sets.

Some ways to use a timer in your isometric exercise routine include:

- Setting a timer for the desired hold time (such as 30 seconds or 1 minute) and maintaining the position until the timer goes off
- Using a stopwatch to track your total hold time for each exercise, and trying to beat your personal record over time
- Setting a timer for your rest periods between sets, ensuring that you're taking enough time to recover but not so much that you lose momentum

When choosing a timer or stopwatch, look for one that is easy to use and read, with clear buttons and a large display. You may also want to choose a model with interval timing or programmable settings for added customization.

## 6. Other Accessories to Consider

In addition to these essential tools, there are a few other accessories you may want to consider adding to your isometric exercise space:

- Wrist wraps or gloves for added support and comfort during plank holds or push-up holds
- A mirror for checking your form and alignment during exercises
- A towel or mat spray for wiping down your equipment and keeping your space clean and hygienic
- A water bottle for staying hydrated during your workouts
- Comfortable, breathable clothing that allows for full range of motion and won't restrict your movements

By investing in a few key pieces of equipment and accessories, you can create a functional and effective isometric exercise space that will support your training goals and help you stay motivated over time.

Remember, the most important thing is to choose tools that work for you and your unique needs and preferences. Don't feel like you need to buy every accessory on the market — start with the essentials and build up your collection over time as your training progresses.

With the right equipment and accessories in place, you'll be well on your way to maximizing the benefits of isometric exercises and achieving your fitness goals. In the next chapter, we'll dive into some fundamental isometric exercises that you can start incorporating into your routine right away. Get ready to feel the burn!

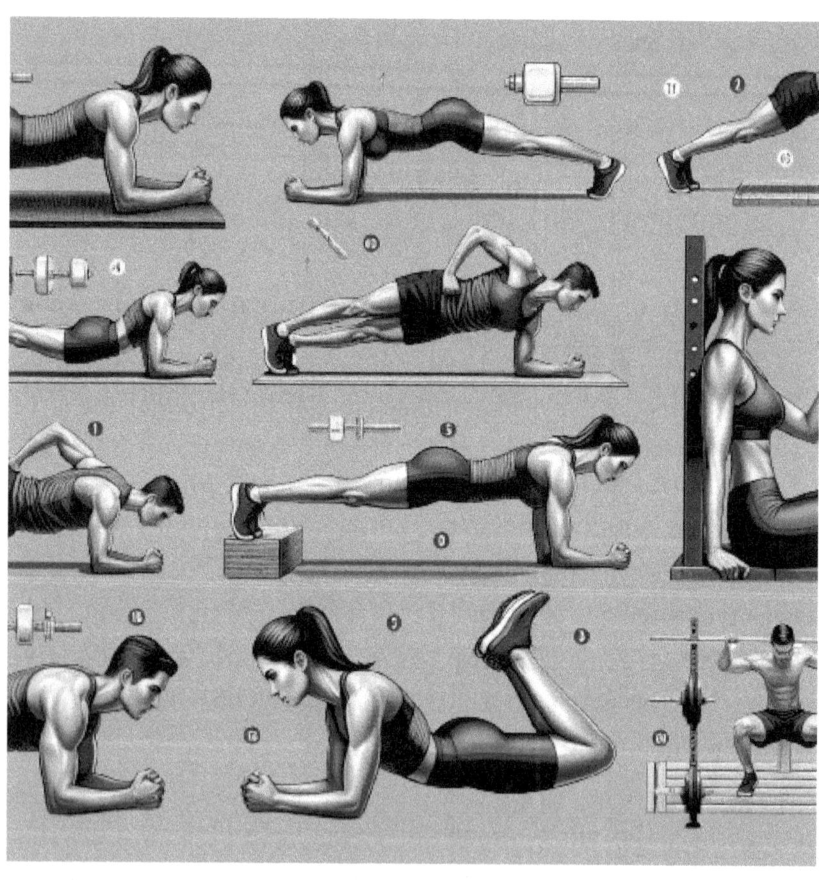

When it comes to fundamental isometric exercises, the plank reigns supreme as the king of core stability. This simple but challenging exercise engages multiple muscle groups simultaneously, helping to build strength, endurance, and stability throughout the entire core region.

Let's take a closer look at the plank exercise and why it's such a valuable addition to your isometric training routine:

## 1. Anatomy of the Plank

The plank primarily targets the core muscles, which include:

- Rectus abdominis: The "six-pack" muscle that runs down the front of your abdomen
- Transverse abdominis: The deepest layer of abdominal muscle that wraps around your spine and helps to stabilize your trunk
- Obliques: The muscles on the sides of your abdomen that help with rotation and lateral flexion

In addition to the core muscles, the plank also engages the:

- Shoulders and upper back: The plank position requires you to stabilize your shoulder blades and engage your upper back muscles to maintain proper form

- Glutes and legs: The plank engages your glutes and leg muscles to help keep your body in a straight line from head to heels

By engaging all of these muscle groups simultaneously, the plank helps to build a strong, stable foundation that can translate to improved performance in other exercises and daily activities.

## 2. Benefits of the Plank

Incorporating the plank into your isometric exercise routine can provide a range of benefits, including:

- Improved core strength and stability: The plank is one of the most effective exercises for targeting the deep abdominal muscles that are critical for maintaining proper posture and stability throughout the spine.

- Better posture: By strengthening the muscles that support your spine, the plank can help to improve your posture and reduce the risk of back pain and injuries.

- Enhanced balance and coordination: The plank requires you to maintain a stable, balanced position while engaging multiple muscle groups simultaneously, which can help to improve your overall balance and coordination.

- Increased muscular endurance: The plank is an endurance exercise that challenges your muscles to work for an extended period, helping to build stamina and endurance over time.

- Versatility and convenience: The plank can be performed anywhere, without any equipment, making it a convenient exercise to incorporate into your routine at home, at the gym, or on the go.

## 3. How to Perform the Plank

To perform a basic plank, follow these steps:

1. Start in a push-up position, with your hands slightly wider than shoulder-width apart and your feet together.

2. Lower your forearms to the ground, so that your elbows are directly under your shoulders and your forearms are parallel to each other.

3. Engage your core muscles and lift your body off the ground, so that you're resting on your forearms and toes.

4. Keep your body in a straight line from head to heels, without letting your hips sag or your back arch.

5. Hold this position for the desired amount of time, focusing on maintaining proper form and breathing steadily throughout the exercise.

As you build strength and endurance, you can gradually increase the duration of your plank holds, working up to longer intervals over time.

## 4. Plank Variations and Progressions

Once you've mastered the basic plank, there are many variations and progressions you can try to keep challenging your muscles and avoid plateaus. Some examples include:

- High plank: Perform the plank with your arms fully extended, as if you were at the top of a push-up position.

- Side plank: Rotate to one side, so that you're resting on one forearm and the side of one foot, with your other arm extended towards the ceiling.

- Plank with leg lift: From the basic plank position, lift one foot off the ground and hold for a few seconds before switching sides.

- Plank with arm lift: From the basic plank position, lift one arm off the ground and extend it in front of you, holding for a few seconds before switching sides.

- Plank walk-outs: Start in a standing position, then walk your hands out into a plank position, hold for a few seconds, then walk your feet back up to your hands to return to standing.

By incorporating these variations and progressions into your routine, you can continue to challenge your muscles and make progress over time.

## 5. Common Plank Mistakes to Avoid

While the plank may seem like a simple exercise, there are a few common mistakes that can compromise its effectiveness and increase the risk of injury. To get the most out of your plank holds, be sure to avoid these mistakes:

- Letting your hips sag: If your hips drop towards the ground, you'll put extra strain on your lower back and reduce the engagement of your core muscles. Keep your body in a straight line throughout the exercise.

- Holding your breath: It's important to breathe steadily throughout your plank holds to ensure that your muscles are getting enough oxygen. Focus on taking deep, even breaths in through your nose and out through your mouth.

- Hunching your shoulders: If you let your shoulders creep up towards your ears, you'll put extra strain on your neck and upper back. Keep your shoulders down and away from your ears, engaging your upper back muscles to maintain proper form.

- Forgetting to engage your glutes: Your glutes play a key role in stabilizing your hips and lower back during the plank. Be sure to squeeze your glutes throughout the exercise to help maintain proper alignment and protect your lower back.

By avoiding these common mistakes and focusing on maintaining proper form, you can maximize the benefits of the plank exercise and reduce the risk of injury.

The plank is a fundamental isometric exercise that should be a staple in every fitness enthusiast's routine. By building core strength, stability, and endurance, the plank can help to improve posture, reduce the risk of injury, and enhance overall athletic performance.

So what are you waiting for? Get down on the ground and start planking! With consistent practice and proper form, you'll be amazed at how quickly you can build a strong, stable core that will support you in all of your fitness endeavors.

Next up, we'll dive into another fundamental isometric exercise: the wall sit. Get ready to feel the burn in your legs and glutes as we explore this classic move and its many variations and progressions.

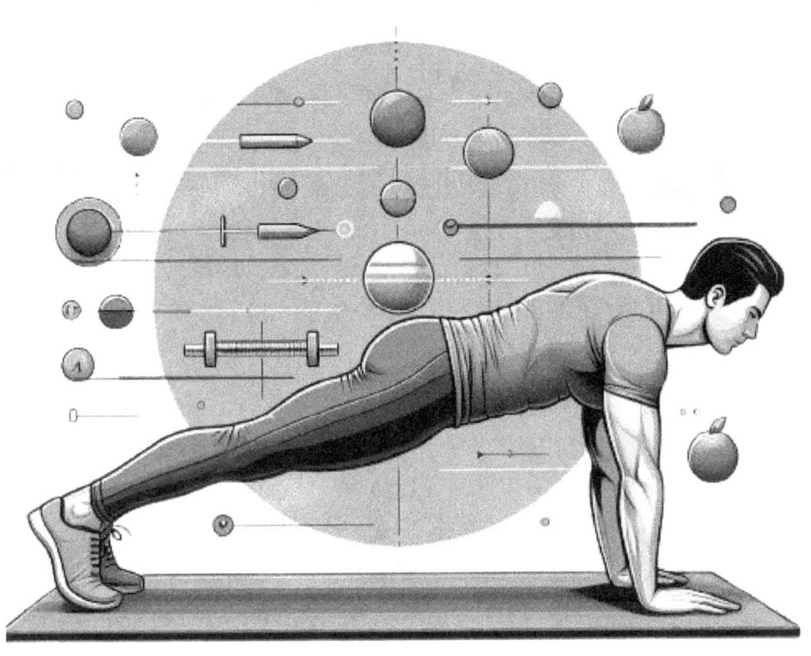

If you're looking to build strong, powerful legs, look no further than the wall sit. This classic isometric exercise is a favorite among athletes, fitness enthusiasts, and anyone looking to sculpt lean, defined legs and glutes.

Let's take a closer look at the wall sit exercise and how it can help you build the legs of your dreams:

## 1. Anatomy of the Wall Sit

The wall sit primarily targets the quadriceps, the large muscle group on the front of your thighs. The quadriceps consist of four individual muscles:

- Rectus femoris: The largest of the quadriceps muscles, which runs down the center of the thigh and helps to extend the knee and flex the hip
- Vastus lateralis: The outer quad muscle that helps to extend the knee and stabilize the kneecap
- Vastus medialis: The inner quad muscle that helps to extend the knee and stabilize the kneecap
- Vastus intermedius: The deep quad muscle that lies beneath the rectus femoris and helps to extend the knee

In addition to the quadriceps, the wall sit also engages the:

- Glutes: The muscles of your buttocks that help to extend the hip and stabilize the pelvis
- Hamstrings: The muscles on the back of your thighs that help to flex the knee and extend the hip

- Calves: The muscles on the back of your lower legs that help to plantarflex the foot (point the toes)

By engaging all of these muscle groups simultaneously, the wall sit helps to build overall leg strength and endurance, while also improving stability and balance.

## 2. Benefits of the Wall Sit

Incorporating the wall sit into your isometric exercise routine can provide a range of benefits, including:

- Increased leg strength and endurance: The wall sit is a highly effective exercise for building strength and endurance in the quadriceps, glutes, and other leg muscles.

- Improved knee stability: By strengthening the muscles around the knee joint, the wall sit can help to improve knee stability and reduce the risk of injury.

- Enhanced athletic performance: Strong, powerful legs are essential for many sports and athletic activities, from running and jumping to skiing and cycling. The wall sit can help to improve your performance in these activities by building the strength and endurance you need to excel.

- Convenience and versatility: Like the plank, the wall sit can be performed anywhere, without any equipment, making it a convenient exercise to incorporate into your routine at home, at the gym, or on the go.

## 3. How to Perform the Wall Sit

To perform a basic wall sit, follow these steps:

1. Start by standing with your back against a wall, with your feet shoulder-width apart and about 2 feet away from the wall.

2. Slowly slide your back down the wall, bending your knees and lowering your hips until your thighs are parallel to the ground (or as close as you can comfortably get).

3. Keep your back flat against the wall, your core engaged, and your hands at your sides or on your thighs.

4. Hold this position for the desired amount of time, focusing on keeping your breathing steady and your form precise.

As you build strength and endurance, you can gradually increase the duration of your wall sits, working up to longer holds over time.

## 4. Wall Sit Variations and Progressions

Once you've mastered the basic wall sit, there are many variations and progressions you can try to keep challenging your muscles and avoid plateaus. Some examples include:

Single-leg wall sit: Perform the wall sit with one foot lifted off the ground, balancing on the other leg.

- Wall sit with bicep curl: Hold a dumbbell in each hand and perform bicep curls while holding the wall sit position.

- Wall sit with overhead press: Hold a dumbbell in each hand and perform overhead presses while holding the wall sit position.

- Wall sit with medicine ball squeeze: Hold a medicine ball between your thighs and squeeze it tightly while holding the wall sit position.

By incorporating these variations and progressions into your routine, you can continue to challenge your leg muscles and make progress over time.

## 5. Common Wall Sit Mistakes to Avoid

While the wall sit may seem like a simple exercise, there are a few common mistakes that can compromise its effectiveness and increase the risk of injury. To get the most out of your wall sits, be sure to avoid these mistakes:

- Letting your knees go past your toes: If your knees extend too far forward, you'll put extra strain on your knee joints and reduce the engagement of your quadriceps. Keep your knees in line with your ankles throughout the exercise.

- Rounding your back: If you let your back round away from the wall, you'll put extra strain on your lower back and reduce the engagement of your core muscles. Keep your back flat against the wall throughout the exercise.

- Holding your breath: As with the plank, it's important to breathe steadily throughout your wall sits to ensure that your muscles are getting enough oxygen. Focus on taking deep, even breaths in through your nose and out through your mouth.

- Letting your hips sag: If you let your hips drop below parallel, you'll put extra strain on your lower back and reduce the engagement of your leg muscles. Keep your hips level with your knees throughout the exercise.

By avoiding these common mistakes and focusing on maintaining proper form, you can maximize the benefits of the wall sit exercise and reduce the risk of injury.

The wall sit is a fundamental isometric exercise that should be a staple in every leg day routine. By building strength, endurance, and stability in your quadriceps, glutes, and other leg muscles, the wall sit can help you sculpt powerful, defined legs that will turn heads and boost your athletic performance.

So what are you waiting for? Find a wall and start sitting! With consistent practice and proper form, you'll be amazed at how quickly you can build the legs of your dreams.

Next up, we'll explore another classic isometric exercise: the push-up hold. Get ready to feel the burn in your chest, shoulders, and arms as we dive into this challenging move and its many variations and progressions.

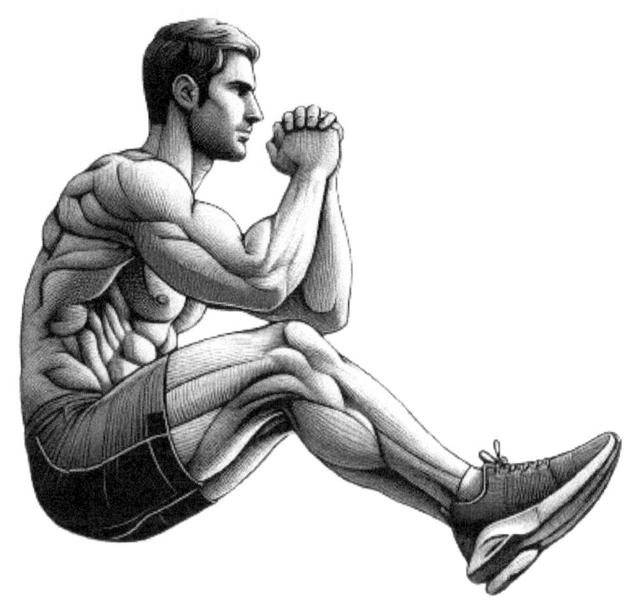

If you're looking to build a strong, powerful upper body, look no further than the push-up hold. This challenging isometric exercise is a favorite among bodybuilders, athletes, and anyone looking to sculpt a chiseled chest, shoulders, and arms.

Let's take a closer look at the push-up hold exercise and how it can help you unleash your upper body strength:

**1. Anatomy of the Push-Up Hold**

The push-up hold primarily targets the chest, shoulders, and triceps, while also engaging the core and back muscles for stability. The main muscles involved in the push-up hold include:

- Pectoralis major: The large chest muscle that helps to horizontally adduct the arm (bring it across the body)
- Deltoids: The shoulder muscles that help to flex and abduct the arm (raise it out to the side)
- Triceps brachii: The muscle on the back of the upper arm that helps to extend the elbow

In addition to these primary movers, the push-up hold also engages the:

- Serratus anterior: The muscle on the side of the ribcage that helps to protract the shoulder blades (pull them forward)

- Rectus abdominis: The "six-pack" muscle that helps to flex the spine and stabilize the core
- Obliques: The muscles on the sides of the waist that help to rotate and laterally flex the spine

By engaging all of these muscle groups simultaneously, the push-up hold helps to build overall upper body strength and stability, while also improving posture and balance.

## 2. Benefits of the Push-Up Hold

Incorporating the push-up hold into your isometric exercise routine can provide a range of benefits, including:

- Increased upper body strength: The push-up hold is a highly effective exercise for building strength in the chest, shoulders, and triceps, which are essential for many upper body movements and activities.

- Improved shoulder stability: By strengthening the muscles around the shoulder joint, the push-up hold can help to improve shoulder stability and reduce the risk of injury.

- Enhanced core strength: The push-up hold requires significant core engagement to maintain proper form and alignment, making it an effective exercise for building overall core strength and stability.

- Increased muscle endurance: By holding the push-up position for an extended period of time, the push-up hold helps to improve muscular endurance, which is essential for activities that require sustained upper body effort, such as climbing or swimming.

### 3. How to Perform the Push-Up Hold

To perform a basic push-up hold, follow these steps:

1. Start in a high plank position, with your hands slightly wider than shoulder-width apart and your feet together.

2. Lower yourself down into a push-up position, with your elbows bent at a 90-degree angle and your chest hovering just above the ground.

3. Hold this position for the desired amount of time, focusing on keeping your core engaged, your back straight, and your breathing steady.

4. Push yourself back up to the starting position, and repeat for the desired number of sets and holds.

As you build strength and endurance, you can gradually increase the duration of your push-up holds, working up to longer holds over time.

### 4. Push-Up Hold Variations and Progressions

Once you've mastered the basic push-up hold, there are many variations and progressions you can try to keep challenging your muscles and avoid plateaus. Some examples include:

- Decline push-up hold: Perform the push-up hold with your feet elevated on a bench or step, which increases the difficulty and targets the upper chest muscles more intensely.

- Single-arm push-up hold: Perform the push-up hold with one hand, while keeping the other hand behind your back or on your hip. This variation increases the challenge and targets each arm individually.

- Push-up hold with shoulder tap: While holding the push-up position, lift one hand off the ground and tap your opposite shoulder, then return to the starting position and repeat on the other side. This variation adds an element of instability and challenges your core and shoulder stability.

- Push-up hold with resistance band: Loop a resistance band around your back and hold the ends in each hand while performing the push-up hold. This variation increases the tension on your chest and triceps muscles, making the exercise more challenging.

By incorporating these variations and progressions into your routine, you can continue to challenge your upper body muscles and make progress over time.

## 5. Common Push-Up Hold Mistakes to Avoid

While the push-up hold may seem like a simple exercise, there are a few common mistakes that can compromise its effectiveness and increase the risk of injury. To get the most out of your push-up holds, be sure to avoid these mistakes:

- Letting your hips sag: If you let your hips drop towards the ground, you'll put extra strain on your lower back and reduce the engagement of your core muscles. Keep your body in a straight line from head to heels throughout the exercise.

- Flaring your elbows: If you let your elbows flare out to the sides, you'll put extra strain on your shoulder joints and reduce the engagement of your chest muscles. Keep your elbows tucked in close to your body throughout the exercise.

- Holding your breath: As with other isometric exercises, it's important to breathe steadily throughout your push-up holds to ensure that your muscles are getting enough oxygen. Focus on taking deep, even breaths in through your nose and out through your mouth.

- Hunching your shoulders: If you let your shoulders creep up towards your ears, you'll put extra strain on your neck and upper back. Keep your shoulders down and away from your ears, engaging your upper back muscles to maintain proper form.

By avoiding these common mistakes and focusing on maintaining proper form, you can maximize the benefits of the push-up hold exercise and reduce the risk of injury.

The push-up hold is a fundamental isometric exercise that should be a staple in every upper body strength routine. By building strength, endurance, and stability in your chest, shoulders, triceps, and core, the push-up hold can help you unleash your full upper body potential and achieve the chiseled, powerful physique you've always wanted.

So what are you waiting for? Drop down and give me a hold! With consistent practice and proper form, you'll be amazed at how quickly you can build the upper body of your dreams.

Next up, we'll explore another classic isometric exercise for the arms: the bicep curl hold. Get ready to feel the burn in your biceps as we dive into this challenging move and its many variations and progressions.

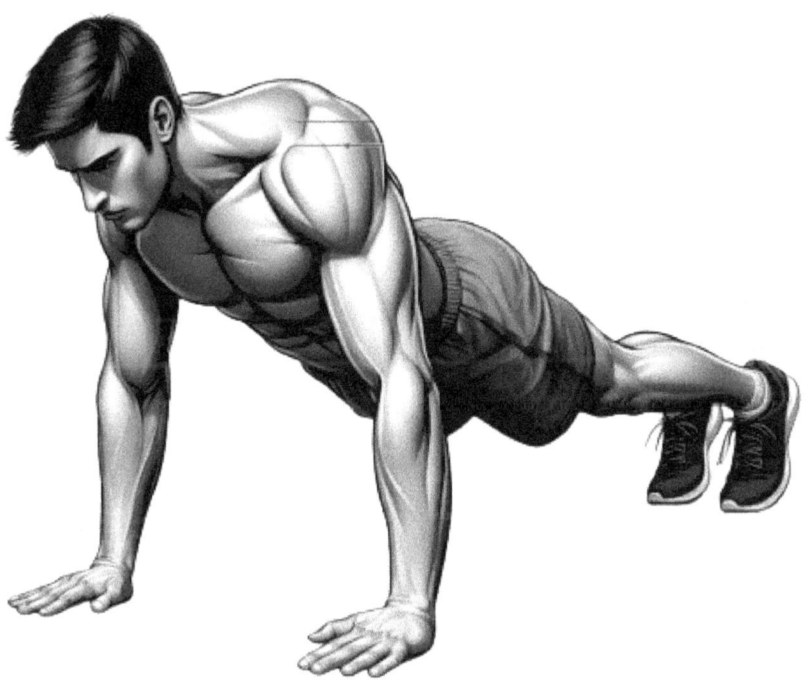

Looking to build a pair of strong, impressive arms? Look no further than the isometric bicep curl. This challenging exercise is a favorite among bodybuilders and fitness enthusiasts alike, and for good reason: it's one of the most effective ways to build strength and size in the biceps muscles.

Let's take a closer look at the isometric bicep curl exercise and how it can help you craft the arms of your dreams:

## 1. Anatomy of the Isometric Bicep Curl

The isometric bicep curl primarily targets the biceps brachii, the large muscle on the front of the upper arm. The biceps brachii has two heads:

- Short head: The inner portion of the biceps muscle that helps to flex the elbow and supinate the forearm (turn the palm upward)
- Long head: The outer portion of the biceps muscle that helps to flex the elbow and supinate the forearm

In addition to the biceps brachii, the isometric bicep curl also engages the:

- Brachialis: The muscle that lies beneath the biceps and helps to flex the elbow
- Brachioradialis: The muscle on the outer forearm that helps to flex the elbow and pronate the forearm (turn the palm downward)

By engaging all of these muscle groups simultaneously, the isometric bicep curl helps to build overall arm strength and size, while also improving grip strength and forearm endurance.

## 2. Benefits of the Isometric Bicep Curl

Incorporating the isometric bicep curl into your arm training routine can provide a range of benefits, including:

- Increased bicep strength: The isometric bicep curl is a highly effective exercise for building strength in the biceps muscles, which are essential for many upper body movements and activities, such as lifting and carrying objects.

- Improved muscle size: By placing the biceps under constant tension, the isometric bicep curl can help to stimulate muscle growth and hypertrophy, leading to larger, more defined biceps over time.

- Enhanced joint stability: By strengthening the muscles around the elbow joint, the isometric bicep curl can help to improve elbow stability and reduce the risk of injury during other upper body exercises and activities.

- Increased grip strength: The isometric bicep curl requires a strong grip to maintain proper form and tension, making it an effective exercise for improving grip strength and forearm endurance.

## 3. How to Perform the Isometric Bicep Curl

To perform a basic isometric bicep curl, follow these steps:

1. Stand with your feet shoulder-width apart and your arms at your sides, holding a dumbbell in each hand with your palms facing forward.

2. Curl the dumbbells up towards your shoulders, keeping your elbows tucked in close to your sides and your upper arms stationary.

3. When your biceps are fully contracted and the dumbbells are at shoulder height, hold this position for the desired amount of time, focusing on maintaining tension in your biceps and keeping your breathing steady.

4. Slowly lower the dumbbells back down to the starting position, and repeat for the desired number of sets and holds.

As you build strength and endurance, you can gradually increase the weight of the dumbbells and the duration of your holds, working up to longer and more challenging sets over time.

## 4. Isometric Bicep Curl Variations and Progressions

Once you've mastered the basic isometric bicep curl, there are many variations and progressions you can try to keep challenging your muscles and avoid plateaus. Some examples include:

- Hammer curl hold: Perform the isometric bicep curl with your palms facing each other, which targets the brachialis and brachioradialis muscles more intensely.

- Preacher curl hold: Perform the isometric bicep curl with your arms resting on a preacher bench, which isolates the biceps muscles and reduces the involvement of other upper body muscles.

- Single-arm bicep curl hold: Perform the isometric bicep curl with one arm at a time, which allows you to focus on each bicep individually and address any strength imbalances between your arms.

- Resistance band bicep curl hold: Perform the isometric bicep curl with a resistance band instead of dumbbells, which provides constant tension throughout the entire range of motion and increases the challenge on your biceps muscles.

By incorporating these variations and progressions into your routine, you can continue to challenge your biceps muscles and make progress towards your arm-building goals.

## 5. Common Isometric Bicep Curl Mistakes to Avoid

While the isometric bicep curl may seem like a simple exercise, there are a few common mistakes that can compromise its effectiveness and increase the risk of injury. To get the most out of your isometric bicep curls, be sure to avoid these mistakes:

- Swinging the weights: If you use momentum to swing the dumbbells up towards your shoulders, you'll reduce the tension on your biceps muscles and increase the risk of injury. Keep your upper arms stationary and focus on contracting your biceps to lift the weights.

- Arching your back: If you arch your back or lean backwards during the exercise, you'll put extra strain on your lower back and reduce the engagement of your biceps muscles. Keep your back straight and your core engaged throughout the movement.

- Holding your breath: As with other isometric exercises, it's important to breathe steadily throughout your bicep curl holds to ensure that your muscles are getting enough oxygen. Focus on taking deep, even breaths in through your nose and out through your mouth.

- Using too much weight: If you use dumbbells that are too heavy for your current strength level, you'll compromise your form and increase the risk of injury. Start with a weight that allows you to maintain proper form throughout the entire hold, and gradually increase the weight as you build strength over time.

By avoiding these common mistakes and focusing on maintaining proper form, you can maximize the benefits of the isometric bicep curl exercise and reduce the risk of injury.

The isometric bicep curl is a powerful exercise for building strong, impressive arms that will turn heads and boost your confidence in and out of the gym. By placing your biceps muscles under constant tension and challenging them to work harder than ever before, the isometric bicep curl can help you unlock your full arm-building potential and achieve the results you've always wanted.

So what are you waiting for? Grab a pair of dumbbells and start curling! With consistent practice and proper form, you'll be amazed at how quickly you can transform your arms and take your physique to the next level.

Next up, we'll explore a challenging isometric exercise for the glutes and hamstrings: the glute bridge hold. Get ready to feel the burn in your backside as we dive into this powerful move and its many variations and progressions.

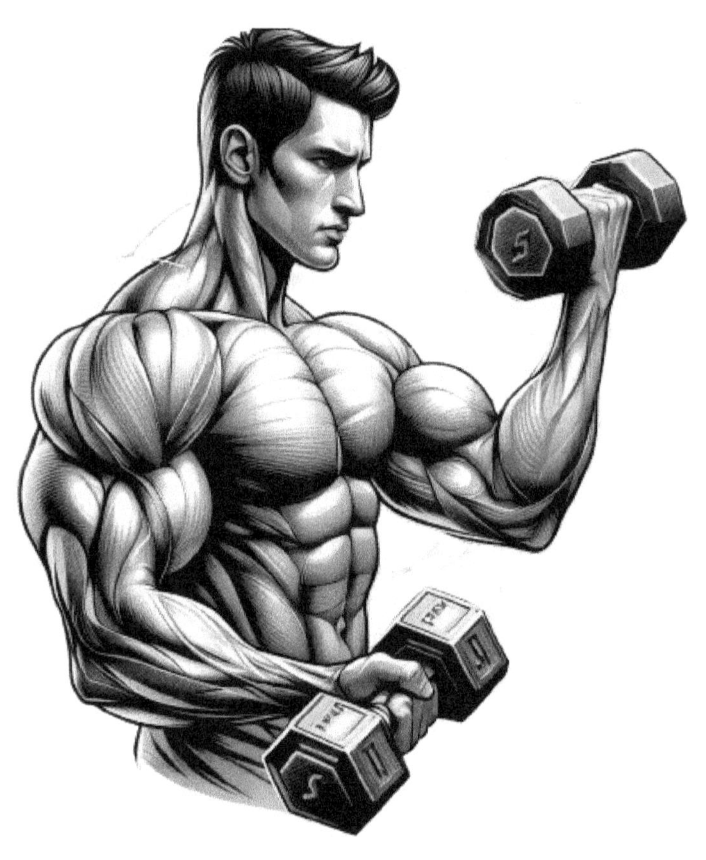

# Glute Bridges: Building a Strong, Resilient Backside

If you're looking to build a strong, powerful backside that can handle anything life throws your way, look no further than the glute bridge. This classic isometric exercise is a favorite among athletes, fitness enthusiasts, and anyone looking to improve their hip and lower back strength and stability.

Let's take a closer look at the glute bridge exercise and how it can help you build a strong, resilient backside:

## 1. Anatomy of the Glute Bridge

The glute bridge primarily targets the gluteus maximus, the largest muscle in the body and the main muscle responsible for hip extension. The gluteus maximus has three main functions:

- Hip extension: Extending the hip joint and moving the thigh backward
- Hip external rotation: Rotating the thigh outward
- Hip abduction: Moving the thigh away from the midline of the body

In addition to the gluteus maximus, the glute bridge also engages the:

- Hamstrings: The muscles on the back of the thigh that help to extend the hip and flex the knee
- Adductors: The muscles on the inner thigh that help to bring the thighs together
- Core muscles: The muscles of the abdomen and lower back that help to stabilize the spine and pelvis

By engaging all of these muscle groups simultaneously, the glute bridge helps to build overall hip and lower back strength and stability, while also improving posture and reducing the risk of injury.

## 2. Benefits of the Glute Bridge

Incorporating the glute bridge into your lower body training routine can provide a range of benefits, including:

- Increased hip strength: The glute bridge is one of the most effective exercises for building strength in the gluteus maximus and other hip muscles, which are essential for many lower body movements and activities, such as walking, running, and jumping.

- Improved lower back health: By strengthening the muscles that support the lower back and pelvis, the glute bridge can help to reduce the risk of lower back pain and injury, and improve overall lower back health and function.

- Enhanced athletic performance: Strong, powerful glutes are essential for many athletic movements and activities, such as sprinting, jumping, and changing direction. The glute bridge can help to improve your performance in these activities by building the strength and power you need to excel.

- Better posture: Weak or underactive glutes can contribute to poor posture and alignment, leading to a host of health problems over time. The glute bridge can help to activate and strengthen the glutes, leading to better posture and alignment throughout the body.

## 3. How to Perform the Glute Bridge

To perform a basic glute bridge, follow these steps:

1. Lie on your back with your knees bent and your feet flat on the ground, hip-width apart.

2. Place your arms at your sides with your palms facing down.

3. Squeeze your glutes and lift your hips off the ground until your body forms a straight line from your knees to your shoulders.

4. Hold this position for the desired amount of time, focusing on maintaining tension in your glutes and keeping your core engaged and your breathing steady.

5. Slowly lower your hips back down to the starting position, and repeat for the desired number of sets and holds.

As you build strength and endurance, you can gradually increase the duration of your holds and the number of sets you perform, working up to longer and more challenging glute bridges over time.

## 4. Glute Bridge Variations and Progressions

Once you've mastered the basic glute bridge, there are many variations and progressions you can try to keep challenging your muscles and avoid plateaus. Some examples include:

- Single-leg glute bridge: Perform the glute bridge with one foot lifted off the ground, which increases the challenge on your glutes and core muscles and helps to address any strength imbalances between your legs.

- Weighted glute bridge: Perform the glute bridge with a weight plate or barbell resting on your hips, which increases the resistance and makes the exercise more challenging.

- Banded glute bridge: Perform the glute bridge with a resistance band around your thighs, just above your knees, which increases the tension on your glutes and hip muscles and makes the exercise more challenging.

- Marching glute bridge: While holding the glute bridge position, lift one foot off the ground and bring your knee towards your chest, then lower it back down and repeat on the other side. This variation adds an element of instability and challenges your balance and coordination.

By incorporating these variations and progressions into your routine, you can continue to challenge your glutes and hip muscles and make progress towards your strength and performance goals.

### 5. Common Glute Bridge Mistakes to Avoid

While the glute bridge may seem like a simple exercise, there are a few common mistakes that can compromise its effectiveness and increase the risk of injury. To get the most out of your glute bridges, be sure to avoid these mistakes:

- Arching your lower back: If you arch your lower back or lift your hips too high during the exercise, you'll put extra strain on your lower back and reduce the engagement of your glutes. Keep your core engaged and your lower back neutral throughout the movement.

- Pushing through your toes: If you push through your toes instead of your heels during the exercise, you'll shift the emphasis away from your glutes and onto your quads and lower back. Keep your weight evenly distributed through your feet and focus on squeezing your glutes to lift your hips.

- Holding your breath: As with other isometric exercises, it's important to breathe steadily throughout your glute bridge holds to ensure that your muscles are getting enough oxygen. Focus on taking deep, even breaths in through your nose and out through your mouth.

- Rushing the movement: If you rush through the exercise or use momentum to lift your hips, you'll reduce the tension on your glutes and hip muscles and increase the risk of injury. Take your time and focus on maintaining tension and control throughout the entire movement.

By avoiding these common mistakes and focusing on maintaining proper form, you can maximize the benefits of the glute bridge exercise and reduce the risk of injury.

The glute bridge is a powerful exercise for building a strong, resilient backside that can handle anything life throws your way. By placing your glutes and hip muscles under constant tension and challenging them to work harder than ever before, the glute bridge can help you unlock your full lower body potential and achieve the strength and performance goals you've always wanted.

So what are you waiting for? Lie down on the floor and start bridging! With consistent practice and proper form, you'll be amazed at how quickly you can transform your backside and take your lower body strength to the next level.

Next up, we'll explore some advanced isometric exercises that will challenge even the most seasoned fitness enthusiasts. Get ready to push your limits and discover what your body is truly capable of!

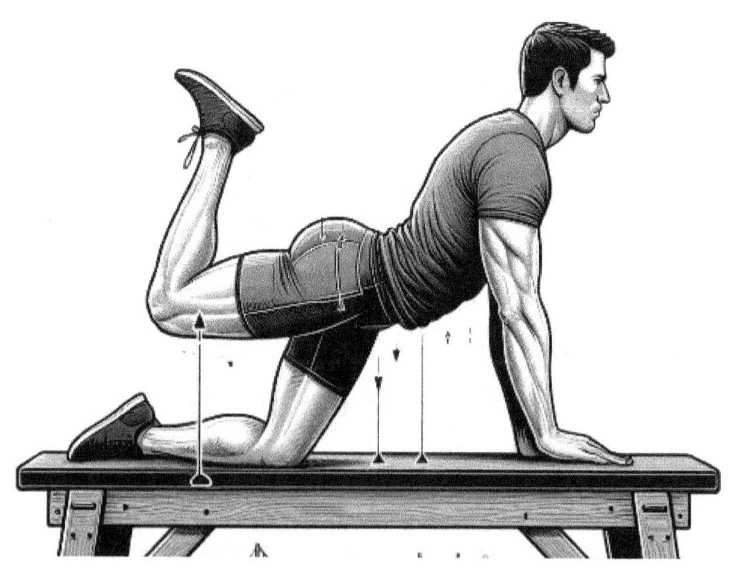

If you're looking to take your upper body strength to the next level and build a powerful, muscular back, look no further than the isometric pull-up. This advanced isometric exercise is a favorite among elite athletes and serious fitness enthusiasts, and for good reason: it's one of the most challenging and effective ways to build strength and control in the back, shoulders, and arms.

Let's take a closer look at the isometric pull-up exercise and how it can help you take back control of your upper body:

**1. Anatomy of the Isometric Pull-Up**
The isometric pull-up primarily targets the latissimus dorsi (lats), the large, flat muscles that run down the sides of your back. The lats have several important functions, including:

- Shoulder extension: Moving the arm down and back from an overhead position
- Shoulder adduction: Bringing the arm down towards the body from an out-to-the-side position
- Shoulder internal rotation: Rotating the arm inward towards the body

In addition to the lats, the isometric pull-up also engages the:

- Trapezius: The large, triangular muscle that runs from the base of the skull to the middle of the back, which helps to elevate and retract the shoulder blades
- Rhomboids: The muscles between the shoulder blades that help to retract and elevate the shoulder blades
- Biceps: The muscles on the front of the upper arm that help to flex the elbow and supinate the forearm
- Core muscles: The muscles of the abdomen and lower back that help to stabilize the spine and pelvis during the exercise

By engaging all of these muscle groups simultaneously, the isometric pull-up helps to build overall upper body strength and control, while also improving posture and reducing the risk of injury.

## 2. Benefits of the Isometric Pull-Up

Incorporating the isometric pull-up into your upper body training routine can provide a range of benefits, including:

- Increased back strength: The isometric pull-up is one of the most effective exercises for building strength in the lats and other back muscles, which are essential for many upper body movements and activities, such as pulling, rowing, and climbing.

- Improved shoulder health: By strengthening the muscles that support the shoulder joint, the isometric pull-up can help to improve shoulder stability and reduce the risk of injury during other upper body exercises and activities.

- Enhanced grip strength: The isometric pull-up requires a strong grip to maintain proper form and tension, making it an effective exercise for improving grip strength and forearm endurance.

- Better posture: Weak or underactive back muscles can contribute to poor posture and a hunched-over appearance. The isometric pull-up can help to strengthen and activate the back muscles, leading to better posture and alignment throughout the upper body.

**3. How to Perform the Isometric Pull-Up**

To perform a basic isometric pull-up, follow these steps:

1. Hang from a pull-up bar with your hands slightly wider than shoulder-width apart and your palms facing away from you.

2. Engage your back muscles and pull yourself up until your chin is above the bar.

3. Hold this position for the desired amount of time, focusing on maintaining tension in your back and keeping your breathing steady.

4. Slowly lower yourself back down to the starting position, and repeat for the desired number of sets and holds.

As you build strength and endurance, you can gradually increase the duration of your holds and the number of sets you perform, working up to longer and more challenging isometric pull-ups over time.

## 4. Isometric Pull-Up Variations and Progressions

Once you've mastered the basic isometric pull-up, there are many variations and progressions you can try to keep challenging your muscles and avoid plateaus. Some examples include:

- Single-arm isometric pull-up: Perform the isometric pull-up with one arm, which increases the challenge on your back and core muscles and helps to address any strength imbalances between your arms.

- Weighted isometric pull-up: Perform the isometric pull-up with a weight belt or weighted vest, which increases the resistance and makes the exercise more challenging.

- Isometric chin-up: Perform the isometric pull-up with your palms facing towards you, which places more emphasis on your biceps and can be a good variation if you have wrist or shoulder issues.

- Towel isometric pull-up: Perform the isometric pull-up while gripping a towel draped over the bar, which increases the challenge on your grip strength and forearm muscles.

By incorporating these variations and progressions into your routine, you can continue to challenge your back and upper body muscles and make progress towards your strength and performance goals.

## 5. Common Isometric Pull-Up Mistakes to Avoid

While the isometric pull-up is a highly effective exercise, there are a few common mistakes that can compromise its effectiveness and increase the risk of injury. To get the most out of your isometric pull-ups, be sure to avoid these mistakes:

- Using momentum: If you use momentum or kipping motions to get your chin above the bar, you'll reduce the tension on your back muscles and increase the risk of injury. Focus on using strict form and engaging your back muscles to pull yourself up.

- Shrugging your shoulders: If you shrug your shoulders up towards your ears during the exercise, you'll reduce the engagement of your lats and other back muscles. Keep your shoulders down and away from your ears throughout the movement.

- Holding your breath: As with other isometric exercises, it's important to breathe steadily throughout your isometric pull-up holds to ensure that your muscles are getting enough oxygen. Focus on taking deep, even breaths in through your nose and out through your mouth.

- Sacrificing form for duration: If you sacrifice proper form in order to hold the isometric pull-up for longer, you'll reduce the effectiveness of the exercise and increase the risk of injury. prioritize proper form and technique over duration, and gradually increase your hold times as you build strength and endurance.

By avoiding these common mistakes and focusing on maintaining proper form and technique, you can maximize the benefits of the isometric pull-up exercise and reduce the risk of injury.

The isometric pull-up is a powerful exercise for building a strong, muscular back and taking your upper body strength to the next level. By placing your back and upper body muscles under constant tension and challenging them to work harder than ever before, the isometric pull-up can help you unlock your full pulling potential and achieve the strength and performance goals you've always wanted.

So what are you waiting for? Grab a pull-up bar and start pulling! With consistent practice and proper form, you'll be amazed at how quickly you can transform your back and take your upper body strength to new heights.

Next up, we'll explore another advanced isometric exercise that will challenge your lower body strength and stability: the single-leg wall sit. Get ready to feel the burn and discover what your legs are truly capable of!

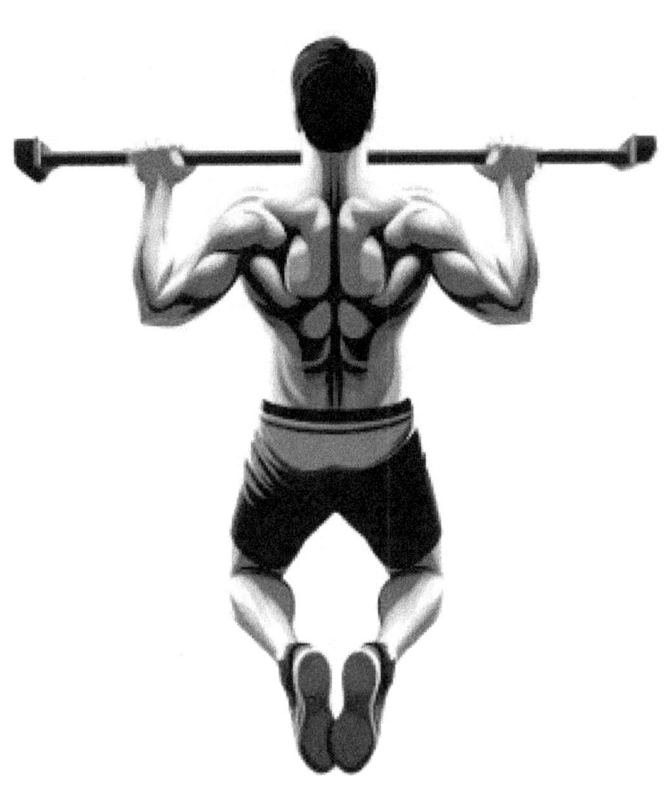

If you're looking to take your lower body strength and stability to the next level, look no further than the single-leg wall sit. This advanced isometric exercise is a favorite among athletes and fitness enthusiasts who want to challenge their legs and core in new and exciting ways.

Let's take a closer look at the single-leg wall sit exercise and how it can help you elevate your lower body game:

## 1. Anatomy of the Single-Leg Wall Sit

The single-leg wall sit primarily targets the quadriceps, the large muscle group on the front of the thigh. The quadriceps consist of four individual muscles:

- Rectus femoris: The largest of the quadriceps muscles, which runs down the center of the thigh and helps to extend the knee and flex the hip
- Vastus lateralis: The outer quad muscle that helps to extend the knee and stabilize the kneecap
- Vastus medialis: The inner quad muscle that helps to extend the knee and stabilize the kneecap
- Vastus intermedius: The deep quad muscle that lies beneath the rectus femoris and helps to extend the knee

In addition to the quadriceps, the single-leg wall sit also engages the:

- Gluteus medius: The muscle on the side of the hip that helps to abduct the leg (move it out to the side) and stabilize the pelvis

- Adductors: The muscles on the inside of the thigh that help to bring the leg back towards the midline of the body
- Hamstrings: The muscles on the back of the thigh that help to flex the knee and extend the hip
- Core muscles: The muscles of the abdomen and lower back that help to stabilize the spine and pelvis during the exercise

By engaging all of these muscle groups simultaneously, the single-leg wall sit helps to build overall lower body strength and stability, while also improving balance and coordination.

## 2. Benefits of the Single-Leg Wall Sit

Incorporating the single-leg wall sit into your lower body training routine can provide a range of benefits, including:

- Increased leg strength: The single-leg wall sit is one of the most effective exercises for building strength in the quadriceps and other leg muscles, which are essential for many lower body movements and activities, such as walking, running, and jumping.

- Improved knee stability: By strengthening the muscles that support the knee joint, particularly the vastus medialis, the single-leg wall sit can help to improve knee stability and reduce the risk of injury.

- Enhanced balance and coordination: The single-leg wall sit requires you to maintain balance and stability on one leg while engaging multiple muscle groups simultaneously, which can help to improve overall balance and coordination.

- Greater core engagement: Because the single-leg wall sit requires you to maintain stability on one leg, it engages the core muscles to a greater extent than the traditional two-legged wall sit, helping to build overall core strength and stability.

**3. How to Perform the Single-Leg Wall Sit**
To perform a basic single-leg wall sit, follow these steps:

1. Stand with your back against a wall, with your feet shoulder-width apart and about 2 feet away from the wall.

2. Slowly slide your back down the wall, bending your knees and lowering your hips until your thighs are parallel to the ground (or as close as you can comfortably get).

3. Lift one foot off the ground and extend that leg out in front of you, keeping your knee straight.

4. Hold this position for the desired amount of time, focusing on keeping your supporting leg engaged and your core tight.

5. Slowly lower your foot back down to the ground, and repeat on the other leg.

As you build strength and endurance, you can gradually increase the duration of your holds and the number of sets you perform, working up to longer and more challenging single-leg wall sits over time.

## 4. Single-Leg Wall Sit Variations and Progressions

Once you've mastered the basic single-leg wall sit, there are many variations and progressions you can try to keep challenging your muscles and avoid plateaus. Some examples include:

- Single-leg wall sit with leg lift: While holding the single-leg wall sit position, lift your extended leg up and down, tapping your toe on the ground each time. This variation adds an element of dynamic movement and increases the challenge on your supporting leg.

- Single-leg wall sit with medicine ball: Hold a medicine ball or other weight in your hands while performing the single-leg wall sit, which increases the overall resistance and engages your upper body and core muscles to a greater extent.

- Single-leg wall sit with hip abduction: While holding the single-leg wall sit position, slowly lift your extended leg out to the side, then lower it back down. This variation targets the gluteus medius and other hip abductor muscles more specifically.

- Single-leg wall sit with knee drive: While holding the single-leg wall sit position, bring your extended leg in towards your chest, then back out to the starting position. This variation engages the hip flexors and core muscles to a greater extent.

By incorporating these variations and progressions into your routine, you can continue to challenge your lower body muscles and make progress towards your strength and performance goals.

**5. Common Single-Leg Wall Sit Mistakes to Avoid**

While the single-leg wall sit is a highly effective exercise, there are a few common mistakes that can compromise its effectiveness and increase the risk of injury. To get the most out of your single-leg wall sits, be sure to avoid these mistakes:

- Letting your knee collapse inward: If you let your supporting knee collapse inward (towards the midline of your body) during the exercise, you'll place extra stress on the knee joint and reduce the engagement of your quadriceps and hip muscles. Keep your knee in line with your hip and ankle throughout the movement.

- Holding your breath: As with other isometric exercises, it's important to breathe steadily throughout your single-leg wall sit holds to ensure that your muscles are getting enough oxygen. Focus on taking deep, even breaths in through your nose and out through your mouth.

- Arching your lower back: If you let your lower back arch away from the wall during the exercise, you'll place extra stress on your lower back and reduce the engagement of your core muscles. Keep your lower back pressed firmly against the wall throughout the movement.

- Letting your hips drop: If you let your hips drop below the level of your knees during the exercise, you'll place extra stress on your knee joint and reduce the engagement of your quadriceps and glutes. Keep your hips level with your knees throughout the movement.

By avoiding these common mistakes and focusing on maintaining proper form and technique, you can maximize the benefits of the single-leg wall sit exercise and reduce the risk of injury.

The single-leg wall sit is a powerful exercise for building lower body strength, stability, and control. By placing your quadriceps, glutes, and core muscles under constant tension and challenging them to work harder than ever before, the single-leg wall sit can help you unlock your full lower body potential and take your performance to the next level.

So what are you waiting for? Find a wall and start sitting! With consistent practice and proper form, you'll be amazed at how quickly you can transform your legs and elevate your lower body game.

Next up, we'll explore another advanced isometric exercise that will challenge your balance, coordination, and overall athleticism: the isometric lunge. Get ready to push your limits and discover what your body is truly capable of!

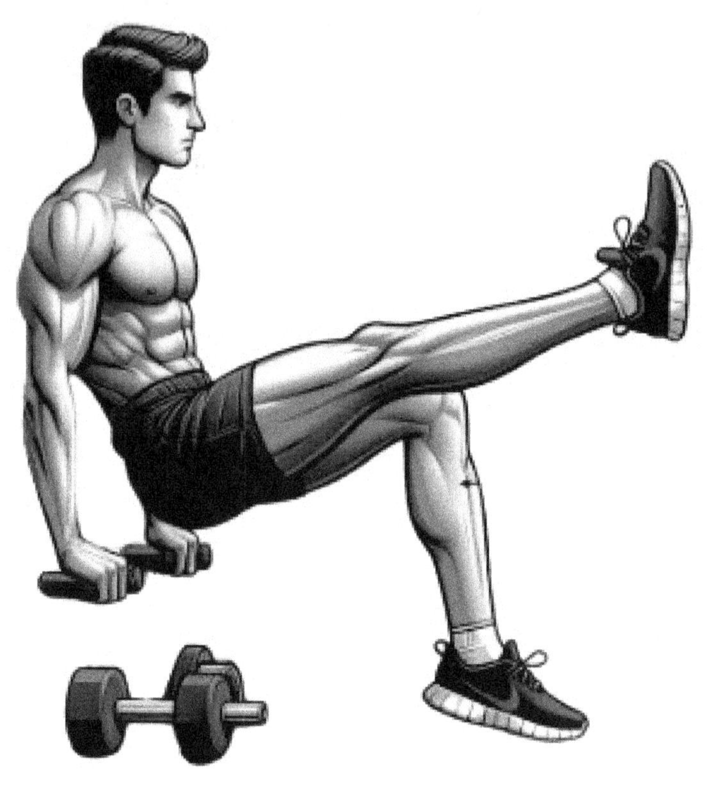

If you're an athlete looking to take your performance to the next level, the isometric lunge is a must-have exercise in your training arsenal. This advanced isometric exercise challenges your balance, coordination, and overall lower body stability, making it an excellent choice for athletes of all kinds.

Let's take a closer look at the isometric lunge exercise and how it can help you develop dynamic stability for peak athletic performance:

## 1. Anatomy of the Isometric Lunge

The isometric lunge is a complex exercise that engages multiple muscle groups throughout the lower body and core. The primary muscles targeted during the isometric lunge include:

- Quadriceps: The large muscle group on the front of the thigh that extends the knee and flexes the hip
- Gluteus maximus: The largest muscle in the body, located in the buttocks, which extends the hip and helps to stabilize the pelvis
- Hamstrings: The muscle group on the back of the thigh that flexes the knee and extends the hip
- Adductors: The muscles on the inside of the thigh that help to bring the leg back towards the midline of the body
- Calves: The muscles on the back of the lower leg that plantarflex the foot (point the toes) and help to stabilize the ankle

In addition to these primary movers, the isometric lunge also engages the core muscles, including the rectus abdominis, obliques, and transverse abdominis, to help stabilize the spine and pelvis during the exercise.

## 2. Benefits of the Isometric Lunge for Athletes

Incorporating the isometric lunge into your athletic training routine can provide a range of benefits, including:

- Improved balance and coordination: The isometric lunge requires you to maintain a stable, balanced position while engaging multiple muscle groups simultaneously, which can help to improve overall balance and coordination, both of which are essential for peak athletic performance.

- Enhanced joint stability: By strengthening the muscles that support the hip, knee, and ankle joints, the isometric lunge can help to improve joint stability and reduce the risk of injury during athletic activities.

- Greater power and explosiveness: The isometric lunge position closely mimics the starting position for many explosive athletic movements, such as sprinting, jumping, and changing direction. By building strength and stability in this position, athletes can improve their power and explosiveness off the line.

- Increased muscular endurance: The isometric lunge is a challenging exercise that requires the lower body muscles to work for an extended period of time under constant tension. This can help to improve muscular endurance, allowing athletes to perform at a high level for longer periods of time

## 3. How to Perform the Isometric Lunge

To perform a basic isometric lunge, follow these steps:

1. Stand with your feet shoulder-width apart and your hands on your hips.

2. Take a large step forward with your right leg, lowering your hips until both knees are bent at a 90-degree angle. Your right knee should be directly over your right ankle, and your left knee should be hovering just above the ground.

3. Hold this position for the desired amount of time, focusing on keeping your core tight, your upper body tall, and your weight evenly distributed between both legs.

4. Push off your right foot to return to the starting position, then repeat on the left leg.

As you build strength and endurance, you can gradually increase the duration of your holds and the number of sets you perform, working up to longer and more challenging isometric lunges over time.

## 4. Isometric Lunge Variations and Progressions

Once you've mastered the basic isometric lunge, there are many variations and progressions you can try to keep challenging your muscles and avoid plateaus. Some examples include:

- Walking isometric lunge: Instead of returning to the starting position after each lunge, step forward with your back leg and immediately lower into another lunge on the opposite side. Continue alternating legs as you walk forward.

- Isometric lunge with overhead press: Hold a dumbbell or other weight in each hand and perform an overhead press while holding the isometric lunge position. This variation engages the upper body and core muscles to a greater extent.

- Isometric lunge with lateral raise: Hold a dumbbell or other weight in each hand and perform a lateral raise (lifting the weights out to the sides) while holding the isometric lunge position. This variation targets the shoulders and upper back muscles.

- Isometric lunge with rotation: While holding the isometric lunge position, rotate your upper body towards the front leg, then back to center. This variation engages the obliques and other core muscles to a greater extent.

By incorporating these variations and progressions into your routine, you can continue to challenge your lower body and core muscles and make progress towards your athletic performance goals.

## 5. Common Isometric Lunge Mistakes to Avoid

While the isometric lunge is a highly effective exercise for athletes, there are a few common mistakes that can compromise its effectiveness and increase the risk of injury. To get the most out of your isometric lunges, be sure to avoid these mistakes:

- Letting your front knee collapse inward: If you let your front knee collapse inward (towards the midline of your body) during the exercise, you'll place extra stress on the knee joint and reduce the engagement of your quadriceps and glute muscles. Keep your knee in line with your hip and ankle throughout the movement.

- Leaning too far forward: If you lean too far forward during the exercise, you'll place extra stress on your lower back and reduce the engagement of your glute and hamstring muscles. Keep your upper body tall and your weight evenly distributed between both legs.

- Holding your breath: As with other isometric exercises, it's important to breathe steadily throughout your isometric lunge holds to ensure that your muscles are getting enough oxygen. Focus on taking deep, even breaths in through your nose and out through your mouth.

- Neglecting proper warm-up: The isometric lunge is a demanding exercise that requires a good deal of mobility and stability in the hips, knees, and ankles. Be sure to perform a proper warm-up before attempting this exercise to reduce the risk of injury.

By avoiding these common mistakes and focusing on maintaining proper form and technique, you can maximize the benefits of the isometric lunge exercise and take your athletic performance to new heights.

The isometric lunge is a powerful exercise for building the dynamic stability and muscular endurance that athletes need to excel in their chosen sports. By placing your lower body and core muscles under constant tension and challenging them to work harder than ever before, the isometric lunge can help you develop the strength, power, and coordination you need to perform at your best.

So what are you waiting for? Find some open space and start lunging! With consistent practice and proper form, you'll be amazed at how quickly you can elevate your athletic performance and take your game to the next level.

Next up, we'll explore an advanced isometric exercise that will challenge your upper body strength, balance, and control: the handstand hold. Get ready to defy gravity and discover what your body is truly capable of!

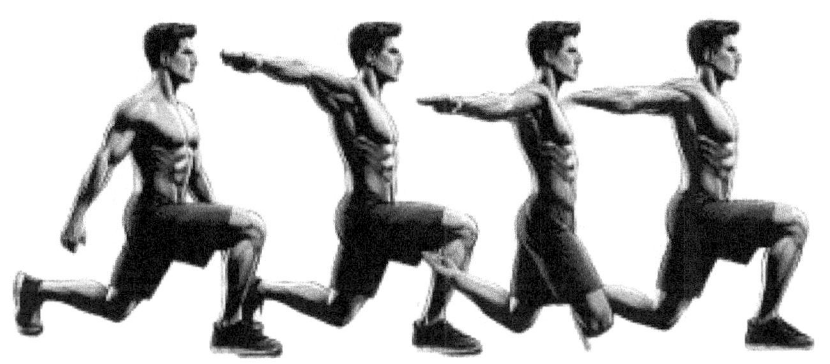

If you're looking for an advanced isometric exercise that will challenge your upper body strength, balance, and control like never before, look no further than the handstand hold. This gravity-defying exercise is a favorite among gymnasts, yogis, and fitness enthusiasts who want to push their bodies to the limit and develop incredible upper body and core strength.

Let's take a closer look at the handstand hold exercise and how it can help you build balance, control, and total-body strength:

## 1. Anatomy of the Handstand Hold

The handstand hold is a complex exercise that engages multiple muscle groups throughout the upper body and core. The primary muscles targeted during the handstand hold include:

- Shoulders: The deltoids, rotator cuff muscles, and other stabilizing muscles of the shoulder girdle work to support the body's weight and maintain proper alignment in the inverted position.

- Triceps: The muscles on the back of the upper arm work to extend the elbow and keep the arms straight during the handstand hold.

- Wrists and forearms: The muscles of the wrists and forearms work to support the body's weight and maintain balance during the handstand hold.

- Core: The rectus abdominis, obliques, and other muscles of the core work to keep the body straight and stable during the handstand hold.

In addition to these primary movers, the handstand hold also engages the muscles of the upper back, chest, and even the legs to some extent, making it a true total-body exercise.

## 2. Benefits of the Handstand Hold

Incorporating the handstand hold into your exercise routine can provide a range of benefits, including:

- Improved upper body strength: The handstand hold is an excellent exercise for building strength in the shoulders, triceps, and other upper body muscles, which can translate to improved performance in other exercises and activities.

- Enhanced balance and body control: The handstand hold requires a great deal of balance and body control to maintain proper alignment and stability in the inverted position. Regularly practicing this exercise can help to improve overall balance and body awareness.

- Greater core stability: The handstand hold engages the core muscles to a high degree to keep the body straight and stable. This can help to improve core strength and stability, which is important for a wide range of athletic and everyday activities.

- Increased confidence and mental toughness: Holding a handstand requires a great deal of mental focus and determination, as well as confidence in one's own abilities. Regularly practicing this exercise can help to build mental toughness and self-confidence that can translate to other areas of life.

### 3. How to Perform the Handstand Hold

To perform a basic handstand hold, follow these steps:

1. Begin by finding a clear, open space near a wall. The wall will serve as a support and safety net as you work on building your handstand hold.

2. Place your hands on the ground about 6 inches away from the wall, with your fingers spread wide and your shoulders directly over your wrists.

3. Kick your legs up and over your head, using the wall for support if needed. Your goal is to find a balanced position with your body in a straight line from head to toe, with your feet together and your toes pointed.

4. Once you find your balance, focus on keeping your core tight, your arms straight, and your breathing steady. Aim to hold the position for a set amount of time, such as 10-30 seconds.

5. When you're ready to come down, tuck your chin to your chest and slowly lower your legs back to the ground, using the wall for support if needed.

As you build strength and confidence, you can gradually work on holding the handstand for longer periods of time and even moving away from the wall for a freestanding hold.

## 4. Handstand Hold Variations and Progressions

Once you've mastered the basic handstand hold, there are many variations and progressions you can try to keep challenging your muscles and advancing your skills. Some examples include:

- Handstand walk: Once you feel comfortable holding a freestanding handstand, try taking small steps forward or backward with your hands, maintaining your balance and alignment as you move.

- Handstand push-up: From the handstand position, slowly lower your head towards the ground by bending your elbows, then push back up to the starting position. This variation adds a dynamic component to the exercise and targets the shoulders and triceps more intensely.

- One-arm handstand hold: For an extra challenge, try holding the handstand position with one arm, keeping the other arm by your side or extended out to the side for balance. This variation requires a great deal of strength and control in the working arm and shoulder.

- Handstand variations on apparatus: If you have access to gymnastic apparatus like parallettes or a yoga trapeze, you can try performing handstand holds and variations using these tools to add an extra element of challenge and instability.

By incorporating these variations and progressions into your routine, you can continue to build upper body strength, balance, and control while keeping your handstand practice fresh and engaging.

## 5. Common Handstand Hold Mistakes to Avoid

While the handstand hold is a highly beneficial exercise, there are a few common mistakes that can hinder progress and increase the risk of injury. To get the most out of your handstand holds, be sure to avoid these mistakes:

- Arching the back: Many people have a tendency to arch their back in the handstand position, which can place excess strain on the lower back and compromise balance. Focus on keeping your core tight and your body in a straight line from head to toe.

- Letting the shoulders collapse: If you let your shoulders collapse towards your ears in the handstand position, you'll place excess strain on the neck and upper back and make it harder to maintain balance. Focus on actively pushing through the shoulders and keeping them away from the ears.

- Forgetting to breathe: As with any isometric exercise, it's important to maintain steady breathing during the handstand hold to ensure that your muscles are getting enough oxygen. Focus on taking slow, deep breaths in through the nose and out through the mouth.

- Rushing the progression: The handstand hold is an advanced exercise that requires a great deal of strength, balance, and body control. Don't rush the progression or attempt variations before you're ready, as this can increase the risk of injury. Take your time and focus on building a solid foundation of strength and technique before moving on to more challenging variations.

By avoiding these common mistakes and focusing on proper form and progression, you can maximize the benefits of the handstand hold exercise and take your upper body strength and control to new heights.

The handstand hold is a powerful and challenging exercise that can help you build incredible upper body strength, balance, and body control. By defying gravity and pushing your body to its limits, the handstand hold can help you develop the confidence, focus, and mental toughness needed to excel in all areas of your fitness journey.

So what are you waiting for? Find a clear space, get inverted, and start holding! With consistent practice and proper form, you'll be amazed at how quickly you can progress and achieve the impressive handstand holds of your dreams.

Next up, we'll explore some sample isometric exercise programs that you can use to start incorporating these powerful exercises into your routine and taking your strength, stability, and control to the next level. Get ready to feel the burn and see the results!

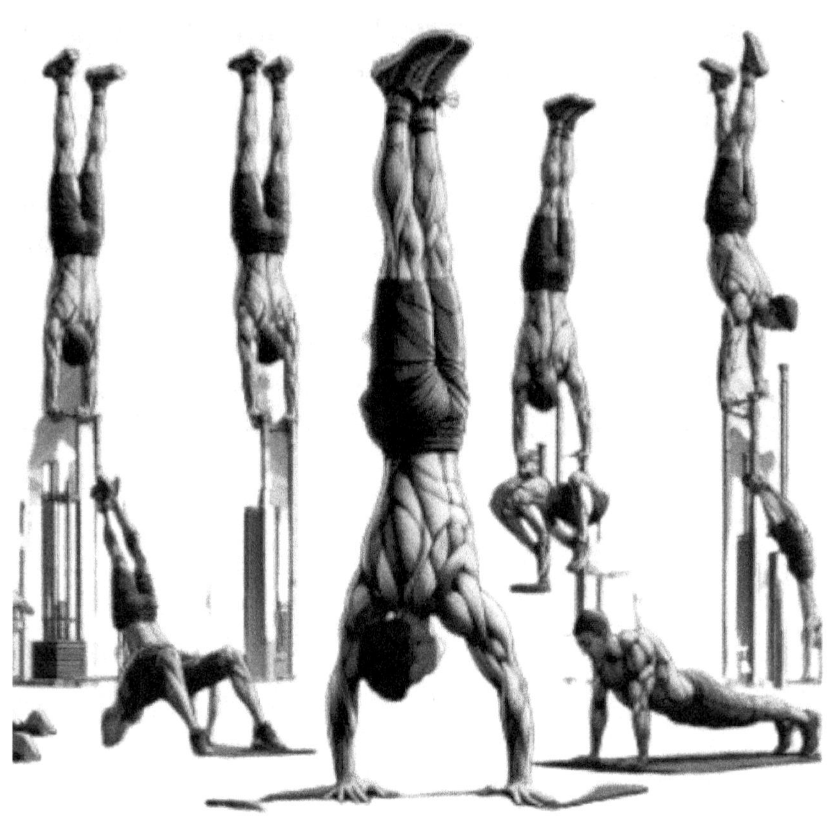

# Chapter 5
## Isometric Exercise Programs

## Beginner's 4-Week Isometric Exercise Program

If you're new to isometric exercises and looking to incorporate them into your fitness routine, a structured program can be a great way to get started and ensure that you're progressing safely and effectively. This beginner's 4-week isometric exercise program is designed to help you build a strong foundation of strength, stability, and body control through a series of basic isometric exercises.

Let's take a closer look at the program and how it can help you get started with isometric training:

## 1. Program Structure
The beginner's 4-week isometric exercise program is divided into four weeks, with three workouts per week. Each workout focuses on a different set of isometric exercises targeting the upper body, lower body, and core muscles.

The workouts are structured as follows:

- Monday: Upper Body Isometrics
- Wednesday: Lower Body Isometrics
- Friday: Core Isometrics

Each workout consists of 3-4 exercises, with each exercise performed for a set number of sets and hold times. The hold times and rest periods between sets will increase gradually over the course of the program to ensure steady progress and adaptation.

## 2. Week 1

In the first week of the program, the focus is on building a base of strength and getting comfortable with the basic isometric exercises. The workouts for Week 1 are as follows:

Monday: Upper Body Isometrics
- Plank Hold: 3 sets of 20-second holds, with 30 seconds rest between sets
- Wall Push-Up Hold: 3 sets of 20-second holds, with 30 seconds rest between sets
- Downward Dog Hold: 3 sets of 20-second holds, with 30 seconds rest between sets

Wednesday: Lower Body Isometrics
- Wall Sit Hold: 3 sets of 20-second holds, with 30 seconds rest between sets
- Single-Leg Balance Hold: 3 sets of 20-second holds per leg, with 30 seconds rest between sets
- Calf Raise Hold: 3 sets of 20-second holds, with 30 seconds rest between sets

Friday: Core Isometrics
- Plank Hold: 3 sets of 20-second holds, with 30 seconds rest between sets
- Side Plank Hold: 3 sets of 20-second holds per side, with 30 seconds rest between sets

- Hollow Body Hold: 3 sets of 20-second holds, with 30 seconds rest between sets

## 3. Week 2

In the second week of the program, the hold times and rest periods are increased slightly to continue challenging the muscles and promoting adaptation. The workouts for Week 2 are as follows:

Monday: Upper Body Isometrics
- Plank Hold: 3 sets of 30-second holds, with 45 seconds rest between sets
- Wall Push-Up Hold: 3 sets of 30-second holds, with 45 seconds rest between sets
- Downward Dog Hold: 3 sets of 30-second holds, with 45 seconds rest between sets

Wednesday: Lower Body Isometrics
- Wall Sit Hold: 3 sets of 30-second holds, with 45 seconds rest between sets
- Single-Leg Balance Hold: 3 sets of 30-second holds per leg, with 45 seconds rest between sets
- Calf Raise Hold: 3 sets of 30-second holds, with 45 seconds rest between sets

Friday: Core Isometrics
- Plank Hold: 3 sets of 30-second holds, with 45 seconds rest between sets
- Side Plank Hold: 3 sets of 30-second holds per side, with 45 seconds rest between sets
- Hollow Body Hold: 3 sets of 30-second holds, with 45 seconds rest between sets

## 4. Week 3

In the third week of the program, a new exercise is introduced for each muscle group to provide a new stimulus and keep the workouts engaging. The workouts for Week 3 are as follows:

Monday: Upper Body Isometrics
- Plank Hold: 3 sets of 40-second holds, with 60 seconds rest between sets
- Eccentric Push-Up Hold: 3 sets of 5 reps with 5-second lowering phase, with 60 seconds rest between sets
- Dolphin Hold: 3 sets of 40-second holds, with 60 seconds rest between sets

Wednesday: Lower Body Isometrics
- Wall Sit Hold: 3 sets of 40-second holds, with 60 seconds rest between sets
- Single-Leg Glute Bridge Hold: 3 sets of 40-second holds per leg, with 60 seconds rest between sets
- Calf Raise Hold: 3 sets of 40-second holds, with 60 seconds rest between sets

Friday: Core Isometrics
- Plank Hold: 3 sets of 40-second holds, with 60 seconds rest between sets
- Side Plank Hold with Leg Lift: 3 sets of 40-second holds per side, with 60 seconds rest between sets
- Hollow Body Rock: 3 sets of 10 reps with 5-second hold at each end, with 60 seconds rest between sets

## 5. Week 4

In the final week of the program, the focus is on pushing the limits and maximizing the challenge to the muscles. The workouts for Week 4 are as follows:

Monday: Upper Body Isometrics
- Plank Hold with Shoulder Taps: 3 sets of 10 reps with 5-second hold per tap, with 75 seconds rest between sets
- Eccentric Push-Up Hold: 3 sets of 8 reps with 8-second lowering phase, with 75 seconds rest between sets
- Dolphin Hold with Leg Lift: 3 sets of 50-second holds per leg, with 75 seconds rest between sets

Wednesday: Lower Body Isometrics
- Wall Sit Hold with Bicep Curls: 3 sets of 50-second holds with 10 bicep curls, with 75 seconds rest between sets
- Single-Leg Glute Bridge Hold with Abduction: 3 sets of 50-second holds per leg with 10 abductions, with 75 seconds rest between sets
- Calf Raise Hold with Toe Taps: 3 sets of 50-second holds with 10 toe taps, with 75 seconds rest between sets

**Friday: Core Isometrics**
- Plank Hold with Knee Tucks: 3 sets of 10 reps with 5-second hold per tuck, with 75 seconds rest between sets
- Side Plank Hold with Rotation: 3 sets of 50-second holds per side with 5 rotations, with 75 seconds rest between sets

- Hollow Body Hold with Toe Taps: 3 sets of 50-second holds with 10 toe taps, with 75 seconds rest between sets

## 6. Progression and Adaptation

By following this 4-week program and gradually increasing the hold times, rest periods, and exercise variations, you can ensure steady progress and adaptation in your isometric strength and endurance.

As you get comfortable with the exercises and your body adapts to the stimulus, you can continue to progress by adding more sets, increasing the hold times, or incorporating more advanced variations of the exercises.

Remember to listen to your body and give yourself adequate rest and recovery between workouts to allow your muscles time to adapt and grow stronger. If you experience any pain or discomfort during the exercises, stop immediately and consult with a qualified fitness professional or healthcare provider.

## 7. Integrating Isometric Exercises into Your Overall Fitness Routine

While this 4-week program is designed to focus specifically on isometric exercises, it's important to remember that isometric training should be just one component of a well-rounded fitness routine.

In addition to isometric exercises, be sure to incorporate other types of training, such as dynamic strength training, cardiovascular exercise, and flexibility work, to ensure balanced development and optimal health and fitness.

You can also use isometric exercises as a supplement to your regular workouts, performing them on off days or as part of your warm-up or cool-down routine to help improve your overall strength, stability, and body control.

The beginner's 4-week isometric exercise program is a great way to get started with isometric training and build a strong foundation of strength, stability, and body control. By following the program consistently and progressively, you can set yourself up for success and lay the groundwork for more advanced isometric training in the future.

So what are you waiting for? Get ready to hold, breathe, and feel the burn as you embark on your isometric training journey and discover the many benefits of this powerful training method. With dedication, consistency, and proper form, you'll be amazed at how quickly you can progress and achieve your fitness goals through isometric exercise.

# Intermediate 6-Week Strength-Building Program

If you've been practicing isometric exercises for a while and are ready to take your strength and endurance to the next level, this intermediate 6-week strength-building program is for you. Designed to challenge your muscles with longer hold times, more advanced exercises, and a greater variety of movements, this program will help you build the strength, power, and stability you need to excel in your fitness journey.

Let's take a closer look at the program and how it can help you achieve your strength-building goals:

## 1. Program Structure

The intermediate 6-week strength-building program is divided into six weeks, with four workouts per week. Each workout focuses on a different set of isometric exercises targeting the upper body, lower body, and core muscles, with an additional full-body workout to integrate all the muscle groups.

The workouts are structured as follows:

- Monday: Upper Body Strength
- Tuesday: Lower Body Strength
- Thursday: Core Strength
- Friday: Full-Body Integration

Each workout consists of 4-5 exercises, with each exercise performed for a set number of sets and hold times. The hold times and rest periods between sets are longer than in the beginner program to provide a greater challenge and stimulus for strength adaptation.

## 2. Week 1-2: Building the Foundation

In the first two weeks of the program, the focus is on building a strong foundation of strength and mastering the proper form and technique for each exercise. The workouts for Weeks 1-2 are as follows:

Monday: Upper Body Strength
- Plank Hold with Arm Lift: 3 sets of 30-second holds per arm, with 60 seconds rest between sets
- Wall Push-Up Hold with Foot Lift: 3 sets of 30-second holds per foot, with 60 seconds rest between sets
- Isometric Bicep Curl Hold: 3 sets of 30-second holds, with 60 seconds rest between sets
- Isometric Tricep Extension Hold: 3 sets of 30-second holds, with 60 seconds rest between sets

Tuesday: Lower Body Strength
- Wall Sit Hold with Calf Raise: 3 sets of 45-second holds with 15 calf raises, with 75 seconds rest between sets
- Single-Leg Squat Hold: 3 sets of 30-second holds per leg, with 60 seconds rest between sets
- Isometric Lunge Hold: 3 sets of 45-second holds per leg, with 75 seconds rest between sets
- Calf Raise Hold with Toe Taps: 3 sets of 45-second holds with 15 toe taps, with 75 seconds rest between sets

Thursday: Core Strength
- Plank Hold with Knee Tucks: 3 sets of 45-second holds with 15 knee tucks, with 75 seconds rest between sets
- Side Plank Hold with Rotation: 3 sets of 45-second holds per side with 10 rotations, with 75 seconds rest between sets
- Hollow Body Hold with Toe Taps: 3 sets of 45-second holds with 15 toe taps, with 75 seconds rest between sets
- Dead Bug Hold: 3 sets of 30-second holds per side, with 60 seconds rest between sets

Friday: Full-Body Integration
- Bear Crawl Hold: 3 sets of 45-second holds, with 75 seconds rest between sets
- Wall Sit Hold with Overhead Press: 3 sets of 45-second holds with 15 presses, with 75 seconds rest between sets
- Plank Hold with Row: 3 sets of 30-second holds per arm with 10 rows, with 60 seconds rest between sets
- Single-Leg Glute Bridge Hold with Curl: 3 sets of 45-second holds per leg with 15 curls, with 75 seconds rest between sets

## 3. Week 3-4: Increasing the Challenge

In the middle two weeks of the program, the focus shifts to increasing the challenge and intensity of the workouts to stimulate further strength adaptation. The workouts for Weeks 3-4 are as follows:

Monday: Upper Body Strength

- Plank Hold with Push-Up: 3 sets of 10 reps with 5-second hold per push-up, with 90 seconds rest between sets
- Handstand Hold Against Wall: 3 sets of 45-second holds, with 75 seconds rest between sets
- Isometric Chin-Up Hold: 3 sets of 30-second holds, with 60 seconds rest between sets
- Isometric Dip Hold: 3 sets of 45-second holds, with 75 seconds rest between sets

Tuesday: Lower Body Strength

- Wall Sit Hold with Single-Leg Extension: 3 sets of 60-second holds with 10 extensions per leg, with 90 seconds rest between sets
- Bulgarian Split Squat Hold: 3 sets of 45-second holds per leg, with 75 seconds rest between sets
- Isometric Lunge Hold with Pulse: 3 sets of 60-second holds per leg with 20 pulses, with 90 seconds rest between sets
- Single-Leg Calf Raise Hold: 3 sets of 45-second holds per leg, with 75 seconds rest between sets

Thursday: Core Strength

- Plank Hold with Shoulder Taps: 3 sets of 60-second holds with 20 taps, with 90 seconds rest between set
- Side Plank Hold with Leg Lift: 3 sets of 60-second holds per side with 10 lifts, with 90 seconds rest between sets
- Hollow Body Hold with Flutter Kicks: 3 sets of 60-second holds with 20 kicks, with 90 seconds rest between sets
- Isometric V-Sit Hold: 3 sets of 45-second holds, with 75 seconds rest between sets

Friday: Full-Body Integration

- Bear Crawl Hold with Shoulder Taps: 3 sets of 60-second holds with 20 taps, with 90 seconds rest between sets
- Wall Sit Hold with Bicep Curl to Overhead Press: 3 sets of 60-second holds with 10 curls to presses, with 90 seconds rest between sets
- Plank Hold with T-Spine Rotation: 3 sets of 45-second holds per side with 10 rotations, with 75 seconds rest between sets
- Single-Leg Glute Bridge Hold with Marching: 3 sets of 60-second holds with 20 marches, with 90 seconds rest between sets

## 4. Week 5-6: Pushing the Limits

In the final two weeks of the program, the focus is on pushing the limits and maximizing the strength and endurance gains. The workouts for Weeks 5-6 are as follows:

Monday: Upper Body Strength

- Plank Hold with Alternating Push-Up: 3 sets of 75-second holds with 10 push-ups per arm, with 105 seconds rest between sets
- Handstand Hold with Shoulder Taps: 3 sets of 60-second holds with 10 taps, with 90 seconds rest between sets
- Isometric Chin-Up Hold with Pulse: 3 sets of 45-second holds with 10 pulses, with 75 seconds rest between sets
- Isometric Dip Hold with Leg Lift: 3 sets of 60-second holds with 10 lifts per leg, with 90 seconds rest between sets

Tuesday: Lower Body Strength

- Wall Sit Hold with Alternating Single-Leg Extension: 3 sets of 75-second holds with 10 extensions per leg, with 105 seconds rest between sets
- Bulgarian Split Squat Hold with Pulse: 3 sets of 60-second holds per leg with 20 pulses, with 90 seconds rest between sets
- Isometric Lunge Hold with Rotation: 3 sets of 75-second holds per leg with 10 rotations, with 105 seconds rest between sets
- Single-Leg Calf Raise Hold with Toe Taps: 3 sets of 60-second holds per leg with 20 taps, with 90 seconds rest between sets

Thursday: Core Strength

- Plank Hold with Push-Up to Knee Tuck: 3 sets of 75-second holds with 10 push-ups to tucks, with 105 seconds rest between sets

- Side Plank Hold with Rotation and Leg Lift: 3 sets of 75-second holds per side with 10 rotations and lifts, with 105 seconds rest between sets
- Hollow Body Hold with Scissor Kicks: 3 sets of 75-second holds with 30 kicks, with 105 seconds rest between sets
- Isometric V-Sit Hold with Twist: 3 sets of 60-second holds with 20 twists, with 90 seconds rest between sets

Friday: Full-Body Integration
- Bear Crawl Hold with Push-Up: 3 sets of 75-second holds with 10 push-ups, with 105 seconds rest between sets
- Wall Sit Hold with Alternating Bicep Curl to Overhead Press: 3 sets of 75-second holds with 10 curls to presses per arm, with 105 seconds rest between sets
- Plank Hold with Row to Rotation: 3 sets of 60-second holds per side with 10 rows to rotations, with 90 seconds rest between sets
- Single-Leg Glute Bridge Hold with Curl to Press: 3 sets of 75-second holds per leg with 10 curls to presses, with 105 seconds rest between sets

## 5. Progression and Adaptation

By following this 6-week program and gradually increasing the hold times, rest periods, and exercise complexity, you can ensure steady progress and adaptation in your isometric strength and endurance.

As you get comfortable with the exercises and your body adapts to the stimulus, you can continue to progress by adding more sets, increasing the hold times, or incorporating even more advanced variations of the exercises.

Remember to listen to your body and give yourself adequate rest and recovery between workouts to allow your muscles time to adapt and grow stronger. If you experience any pain or discomfort during the exercises, stop immediately and consult with a qualified fitness professional or healthcare provider.

## 6. Integrating Isometric Exercises into Your Overall Fitness Routine

As with the beginner program, it's important to remember that isometric training should be just one component of a well-rounded fitness routine.

In addition to isometric exercises, be sure to incorporate other types of training, such as dynamic strength training, cardiovascular exercise, and flexibility work, to ensure balanced development and optimal health and fitness.

You can also use isometric exercises as a supplement to your regular workouts, performing them on off days or as part of your warm-up or cool-down routine to help improve your overall strength, stability, and body control.

The intermediate 6-week strength-building program is a great way to take your isometric training to the next level and challenge your muscles in new and exciting ways. By following the program consistently and progressively, you can build the strength, power, and stability you need to excel in your fitness journey and achieve your goals.

So what are you waiting for? Get ready to hold strong, breathe deep, and embrace the challenge as you embark on this exciting phase of your isometric training journey. With dedication, consistency, and proper form, you'll be amazed at how quickly you can progress and achieve new levels of strength and performance through isometric exercise. Let's do this!

If you've mastered the intermediate isometric training program and are ready to take your physique to the next level, this advanced 8-week muscle sculpting program is for you. Designed to challenge your muscles with intense, targeted isometric contractions and minimal rest periods, this program will help you build dense, defined muscle mass and achieve the sculpted physique you've always wanted.

Let's take a closer look at the program and how it can help you achieve your muscle-sculpting goals:

## 1. Program Structure

The advanced 8-week muscle sculpting program is divided into eight weeks, with five workouts per week. Each workout focuses on a specific muscle group, with an additional full-body workout to integrate all the muscle groups and promote overall muscle balance and symmetry.

The workouts are structured as follows:

- Monday: Chest and Triceps
- Tuesday: Back and Biceps
- Wednesday: Legs and Glutes
- Thursday: Shoulders and Abs
- Friday: Full-Body Integration

Each workout consists of 4-6 exercises, with each exercise performed for a set number of sets and hold times. The hold times are shorter than in the intermediate program, but the intensity is higher, with more advanced exercise variations and shorter rest periods between sets.

## 2. Week 1-2: Acclimation Phase

In the first two weeks of the program, the focus is on acclimating your body to the high-intensity isometric contractions and building a foundation for the muscle-sculpting phase to come. The workouts for Weeks 1-2 are as follows:

Monday: Chest and Triceps
- Isometric Push-Up Hold (narrow grip): 4 sets of 20-second holds, with 40 seconds rest between sets
- Isometric Chest Fly Hold: 4 sets of 30-second holds, with 60 seconds rest between sets
- Isometric Tricep Extension Hold (single arm): 4 sets of 20-second holds per arm, with 40 seconds rest between sets
- Isometric Dip Hold: 4 sets of 30-second holds, with 60 seconds rest between sets

Tuesday: Back and Biceps
- Isometric Pull-Up Hold (wide grip): 4 sets of 20-second holds, with 40 seconds rest between sets
- Isometric Bent-Over Row Hold: 4 sets of 30-second holds, with 60 seconds rest between sets
- Isometric Bicep Curl Hold (hammer grip): 4 sets of 20-second holds per arm, with 40 seconds rest between sets

- Isometric Chin-Up Hold: 4 sets of 30-second holds, with 60 seconds rest between sets

Wednesday: Legs and Glutes
- Isometric Squat Hold: 4 sets of 45-second holds, with 75 seconds rest between sets
- Isometric Lunge Hold (split stance): 4 sets of 30-second holds per leg, with 60 seconds rest between sets
- Isometric Glute Bridge Hold (single leg): 4 sets of 45-second holds per leg, with 75 seconds rest between sets
- Isometric Calf Raise Hold: 4 sets of 30-second holds, with 60 seconds rest between sets

Thursday: Shoulders and Abs
- Isometric Handstand Hold: 4 sets of 30-second holds, with 60 seconds rest between sets
- Isometric Lateral Raise Hold: 4 sets of 20-second holds per arm, with 40 seconds rest between sets
- Isometric Front Raise Hold: 4 sets of 20-second holds per arm, with 40 seconds rest between sets
- Isometric Plank Hold: 4 sets of 60-second holds, with 90 seconds rest between sets
- Isometric Hollow Body Hold: 4 sets of 45-second holds, with 75 seconds rest between sets

Friday: Full-Body Integration
- Isometric Bear Crawl Hold: 4 sets of 45-second holds, with 75 seconds rest between sets
- Isometric Single-Arm Plank Hold: 4 sets of 30-second holds per arm, with 60 seconds rest between sets

- Isometric Single-Leg Wall Sit Hold: 4 sets of 45-second holds per leg, with 75 seconds rest between sets
- Isometric Burpee Hold (bottom position): 4 sets of 30-second holds, with 60 seconds rest between sets
- Isometric Hollow Body Rock Hold: 4 sets of 45-second holds, with 75 seconds rest between sets

## 3. Week 3-5: Muscle-Sculpting Phase

In the middle three weeks of the program, the focus shifts to maximizing muscle tension and metabolic stress to stimulate muscle growth and definition. The workouts for Weeks 3-5 are as follows:

Monday: Chest and Triceps
- Isometric Push-Up Hold (diamond grip): 5 sets of 15-second holds, with 30 seconds rest between sets
- Isometric Single-Arm Chest Fly Hold: 5 sets of 20-second holds per arm, with 40 seconds rest between sets
- Isometric Tricep Kickback Hold: 5 sets of 15-second holds per arm, with 30 seconds rest between sets
- Isometric Close-Grip Bench Press Hold: 5 sets of 20-second holds, with 40 seconds rest between sets

Tuesday: Back and Biceps
- Isometric Pull-Up Hold (close grip): 5 sets of 15-second holds, with 30 seconds rest between sets
- Isometric Single-Arm Bent-Over Row Hold: 5 sets of 20-second holds per arm, with 40 seconds rest between sets
- Isometric Preacher Curl Hold: 5 sets of 15-second holds per arm, with 30 seconds rest between sets

- Isometric Chin-Up Hold (reverse grip): 5 sets of 20-second holds, with 40 seconds rest between sets

Wednesday: Legs and Glutes
- Isometric Sumo Squat Hold: 5 sets of 30-second holds, with 60 seconds rest between sets
- Isometric Bulgarian Split Squat Hold: 5 sets of 20-second holds per leg, with 40 seconds rest between sets
- Isometric Single-Leg Deadlift Hold: 5 sets of 30-second holds per leg, with 60 seconds rest between sets
- Isometric Donkey Calf Raise Hold: 5 sets of 20-second holds, with 40 seconds rest between sets

Thursday: Shoulders and Abs
- Isometric Handstand Push-Up Hold: 5 sets of 15-second holds, with 30 seconds rest between sets
- Isometric Single-Arm Lateral Raise Hold: 5 sets of 15-second holds per arm, with 30 seconds rest between sets
- Isometric Single-Arm Front Raise Hold: 5 sets of 15-second holds per arm, with 30 seconds rest between sets
- Isometric Plank Hold with Shoulder Taps: 5 sets of 30-second holds with 10 taps, with 60 seconds rest between sets
- Isometric V-Sit Hold: 5 sets of 30-second holds, with 60 seconds rest between sets

**Friday: Full-Body Integration**
- Isometric Bear Crawl Hold with Push-Ups: 5 sets of 30-second holds with 5 push-ups, with 60 seconds rest between sets

- Isometric Single-Arm Plank Hold with Row: 5 sets of 20-second holds per arm with 5 rows, with 40 seconds rest between sets
- Isometric Single-Leg Wall Sit Hold with Bicep Curl: 5 sets of 30-second holds per leg with 5 curls, with 60 seconds rest between sets
- Isometric Burpee Hold with Shoulder Press: 5 sets of 20-second holds with 5 presses, with 40 seconds rest between sets
- Isometric Hollow Body Hold with Twists: 5 sets of 30-second holds with 10 twists, with 60 seconds rest between sets

## 4. Week 6-8: Peak Contraction Phase

In the final three weeks of the program, the focus is on maximizing muscle activation and peak contraction to sculpt and define the muscles. The workouts for Weeks 6-8 are as follows:

Monday: Chest and Triceps
- Isometric Push-Up Hold with 1.5 Reps: 6 sets of 10-second holds with 1.5 reps, with 20 seconds rest between sets
- Isometric Cable Crossover Hold: 6 sets of 15-second holds per arm, with 30 seconds rest between sets
- Isometric Tricep Extension Hold with Pulse: 6 sets of 10-second holds with 5 pulses per arm, with 20 seconds rest between sets
- Isometric Dip Hold with Knee Raise: 6 sets of 15-second holds with 5 knee raises, with 30 seconds rest between sets

Tuesday: Back and Biceps

- Isometric Pull-Up Hold with 1.5 Reps: 6 sets of 10-second holds with 1.5 reps, with 20 seconds rest between sets
- Isometric Single-Arm Cable Row Hold: 6 sets of 15-second holds per arm, with 30 seconds rest between sets
- Isometric Bicep Curl Hold with Pulse: 6 sets of 10-second holds with 5 pulses per arm, with 20 seconds rest between sets
- Isometric Chin-Up Hold with Leg Raise: 6 sets of 15-second holds with 5 leg raises, with 30 seconds rest between sets

Wednesday: Legs and Glutes

- Isometric Squat Hold with Pulse: 6 sets of 20-second holds with 10 pulses, with 40 seconds rest between sets
- Isometric Reverse Lunge Hold with Knee Drive: 6 sets of 15-second holds per leg with 5 knee drives, with 30 seconds rest between sets
- Isometric Single-Leg Hip Thrust Hold with Abduction: 6 sets of 20-second holds per leg with 10 abductions, with 40 seconds rest between sets
- Isometric Single-Leg Calf Raise Hold with Bounce: 6 sets of 15-second holds per leg with 10 bounces, with 30 seconds rest between sets

Thursday: Shoulders and Abs

- Isometric Pike Push-Up Hold: 6 sets of 10-second holds, with 20 seconds rest between sets
- Isometric Lateral Raise Hold with Pulse: 6 sets of 10-second holds per arm with 5 pulses, with 20 seconds rest between sets

- Isometric Front Raise Hold with Rotation: 6 sets of 10-second holds per arm with 5 rotations, with 20 seconds rest between sets
- Isometric Plank Hold with Knee Drive: 6 sets of 20-second holds with 10 knee drives, with 40 seconds rest between sets
- Isometric Hollow Body Hold with Scissors: 6 sets of 20-second holds with 10 scissors, with 40 seconds rest between sets

Friday: Full-Body Integration
- Isometric Bear Plank Hold with Shoulder Tap and Knee Drive: 6 sets of 20-second holds with 5 taps and drives, with 40 seconds rest between sets
- Isometric Single-Arm Plank Hold with Row and Kick: 6 sets of 15-second holds per arm with 5 rows and kicks, with 30 seconds rest between sets
- Isometric Single-Leg Wall Sit Hold with Overhead Press: 6 sets of 20-second holds per leg with 10 presses, with 40 seconds rest between sets
- Isometric Burpee Hold with Push-Up and Jump: 6 sets of 15-second holds with 1 push-up and jump, with 30 seconds rest between sets
- Isometric Hollow Body Hold with Flutter Kick: 6 sets of 20-second holds with 20 kicks, with 40 seconds rest between sets

## 5. Progression and Adaptation

By following this 8-week program and gradually increasing the intensity, volume, and complexity of the exercises, you can ensure maximal muscle stimulation and adaptation.

As you get stronger and more comfortable with the exercises, you can continue to progress by adding more sets, decreasing the rest periods, or incorporating even more advanced exercise variations and techniques, such as drop sets, supersets, and pyramid sets.

Remember to listen to your body and give yourself adequate rest and recovery between workouts to allow your muscles time to grow and adapt. If you experience any pain or discomfort during the exercises, stop immediately and consult with a qualified fitness professional or healthcare provider.

## 6. Nutrition and Supplementation

To maximize muscle growth and definition, it's important to support your isometric training with a balanced, nutrient-dense diet and appropriate supplementation.

Aim to consume a diet that is high in lean protein, complex carbohydrates, and healthy fats, with a focus on whole, minimally processed foods. Consider tracking your macronutrient intake to ensure that you are consuming enough protein to support muscle growth and repair, as well as enough carbohydrates to fuel your workouts and replenish glycogen stores.

In terms of supplementation, consider incorporating a high-quality protein powder, creatine monohydrate, and branched-chain amino acids (BCAAs) into your routine to support muscle growth, strength, and recovery. Be sure to consult with a qualified healthcare provider before starting any new supplement regimen.

## 7. Rest and Recovery

Adequate rest and recovery are essential for maximizing muscle growth and preventing overtraining and injury. Aim to get at least 7-9 hours of quality sleep per night, and incorporate active recovery techniques such as foam rolling, stretching, and massage into your routine.

Consider taking 1-2 rest days per week, or alternating between high-intensity isometric training days and lower-intensity cardio or mobility days to allow your muscles time to recover and adapt.

The advanced 8-week muscle sculpting program is a challenging but highly effective way to take your physique to the next level and achieve the dense, defined muscle mass you've always wanted. By following the program consistently and supporting your training with proper nutrition, supplementation, and recovery techniques, you can maximize your results and achieve your best body yet.

So what are you waiting for? Get ready to embrace the challenge, push your limits, and sculpt the physique of your dreams with this advanced isometric training program. Remember, consistency is key, and with hard work and dedication, anything is possible. Let's get started!

## Running

Running is a high-impact, full-body activity that requires strength, endurance, and stability in multiple muscle groups. Incorporating isometric exercises into your running training can help improve your performance, reduce your risk of injury, and enhance your overall running efficiency.

Let's take a closer look at how isometric exercises can benefit runners and some specific exercises to incorporate into your training routine:

### 1. Benefits of Isometric Exercises for Runners

Isometric exercises offer several key benefits for runners, including:

- Improved running economy: Isometric exercises can help improve your running economy, or the amount of energy you expend while running at a given pace. By strengthening key muscle groups and improving your ability to generate and maintain force, isometric exercises can help you run more efficiently and with less effort.

- Increased muscular endurance: Running requires a high level of muscular endurance, particularly in the legs and core. Isometric exercises can help build the endurance you need to maintain proper form and technique throughout long runs and races.

- Enhanced joint stability: Running places a significant amount of stress on the joints, particularly the ankles, knees, and hips. Isometric exercises can help strengthen the muscles and connective tissues around these joints, improving stability and reducing the risk of injury.

- Greater core strength: A strong, stable core is essential for maintaining proper running form and transferring power between the upper and lower body. Isometric exercises that target the core, such as planks and hollow holds, can help improve your running posture and efficiency.

## 2. Key Muscle Groups for Runners

When incorporating isometric exercises into your running training, it's important to focus on the key muscle groups that are most important for running performance and injury prevention. These include:

- Glutes: The gluteal muscles, particularly the gluteus maximus, are responsible for extending the hip and propelling the body forward during running. Weak or underactive glutes can lead to poor running form and increased risk of injury.

- Quadriceps: The quadriceps muscles, located on the front of the thigh, are responsible for extending the knee and absorbing impact during running. Strong quads are essential for maintaining proper running form and preventing knee injuries.

- Hamstrings: The hamstring muscles, located on the back of the thigh, work in conjunction with the glutes to extend the hip and flex the knee during running. Strong, flexible hamstrings are important for preventing muscle strains and other injuries.

- Calves: The calf muscles, particularly the gastrocnemius and soleus, are responsible for plantarflexing the foot and propelling the body forward during running. Strong, resilient calves are important for maintaining ankle stability and preventing Achilles tendon injuries.

- Core: The core muscles, including the rectus abdominis, obliques, and transverse abdominis, are responsible for maintaining proper running posture and transferring power between the upper and lower body. A strong, stable core is essential for efficient running and injury prevention.

### 3. Isometric Exercises for Runners

Here are some specific isometric exercises that can benefit runners:

- Isometric Single-Leg Glute Bridge: Lie on your back with one foot flat on the ground and the other leg extended straight up toward the ceiling. Push through your heel to lift your hips off the ground, holding for 30-60 seconds per side. This exercise targets the glutes and hamstrings.

- Isometric Split Squat: Stand with one foot elevated on a bench or step behind you, with your front leg bent at a 90-degree angle. Lower your back knee toward the ground, holding for 30-60 seconds per side. This exercise targets the quads, glutes, and hamstrings.

- Isometric Calf Raise: Stand with the balls of your feet on the edge of a step or platform, with your heels hanging off the edge. Rise up onto your toes, holding for 30-60 seconds. This exercise targets the calves.

- Isometric Plank: Start in a push-up position, with your forearms on the ground and your elbows directly under your shoulders. Keep your body in a straight line from head to heels, holding for 30-60 seconds. This exercise targets the core and upper body.

- Isometric Single-Leg Wall Sit: Stand with your back against a wall and one foot elevated off the ground. Lower your hips until your knee is bent at a 90-degree angle, holding for 30-60 seconds per side. This exercise targets the quads and glutes.

## 4. Incorporating Isometric Exercises into Your Running Routine

To get the most benefit from isometric exercises, it's important to incorporate them into your running routine in a strategic way. Here are some tips:

- Perform isometric exercises 2-3 times per week, on non-running days or after easy runs.

- Start with shorter hold times (10-20 seconds) and gradually progress to longer holds (30-60 seconds) as you build strength and endurance.
- Focus on maintaining proper form and alignment throughout each exercise, engaging the targeted muscle groups and avoiding compensatory movements.
- Pair isometric exercises with dynamic stretching and mobility work to maintain flexibility and range of motion.
- Listen to your body and adjust your training as needed to avoid overuse injuries or excessive fatigue.

## 5. Sample Isometric Workout for Runners

Here's a sample isometric workout that targets the key muscle groups for running:

1. Isometric Single-Leg Glute Bridge: 3 sets of 30-second holds per leg
2. Isometric Split Squat: 3 sets of 45-second holds per leg
3. Isometric Calf Raise: 3 sets of 60-second holds
4. Isometric Plank: 3 sets of 60-second holds
5. Isometric Single-Leg Wall Sit: 3 sets of 45-second holds per leg

Perform this workout 2-3 times per week, allowing for adequate rest and recovery between sessions.

## 6. Precautions and Considerations

While isometric exercises can be highly beneficial for runners, there are some precautions and considerations to keep in mind:

- If you have a history of high blood pressure or cardiovascular disease, consult with your doctor before starting an isometric exercise program.
- If you experience pain or discomfort during any exercise, stop immediately and seek medical attention if necessary.
- Avoid holding your breath during isometric exercises, as this can cause a sudden spike in blood pressure. Focus on maintaining steady, controlled breathing throughout each hold.
- Don't neglect other aspects of your running training, such as cardiovascular endurance, flexibility, and dynamic strength work. Isometric exercises should be one component of a well-rounded training program.

Incorporating isometric exercises into your running routine can help you build the strength, endurance, and stability you need to perform your best and stay injury-free. By targeting key muscle groups and maintaining proper form and technique, you can enhance your running efficiency and enjoyment for years to come.

So what are you waiting for? Start adding isometric exercises to your running training today, and see the difference they can make in your performance and overall health. Remember, consistency is key, and even small changes can lead to big improvements over time. Happy running!

# Swimming

Swimming is a low-impact, full-body activity that requires a unique combination of strength, endurance, and technique. Incorporating isometric exercises into your swim training can help improve your performance, increase your power output, and reduce your risk of injury.

Let's dive into how isometric exercises can benefit swimmers and explore some specific exercises to incorporate into your training routine:

**1. Benefits of Isometric Exercises for Swimmers**
Isometric exercises offer several key benefits for swimmers, including:

- Increased power output: Swimming requires explosive power, particularly during starts, turns, and sprint events. Isometric exercises can help build the strength and power you need to generate maximum force in the water.

- Improved core stability: A strong, stable core is essential for maintaining proper body position and alignment in the water. Isometric exercises that target the core, such as planks and hollow holds, can help improve your swimming posture and efficiency.

- Enhanced shoulder stability: Swimming places a significant amount of stress on the shoulder joint, particularly during overhead movements like the freestyle and butterfly strokes.

- Isometric exercises can help strengthen the muscles and connective tissues around the shoulder, reducing the risk of overuse injuries.

- Greater hip and leg strength: Strong hips and legs are essential for generating propulsive force in the water, particularly during kicking movements. Isometric exercises that target the glutes, quads, and hamstrings can help improve your kicking power and efficiency.

## 2. Key Muscle Groups for Swimmers

When incorporating isometric exercises into your swim training, it's important to focus on the key muscle groups that are most important for swimming performance and injury prevention. These include:

- Shoulders: The shoulder muscles, particularly the rotator cuff and deltoids, are responsible for generating power and maintaining proper technique during overhead swimming movements. Strong, stable shoulders are essential for preventing overuse injuries like swimmer's shoulder.

- Lats: The latissimus dorsi, or lats, are the large, flat muscles on either side of the back that are responsible for pulling the body through the water during swimming. Strong lats are essential for generating propulsive force and maintaining proper body position in the water.

- Core: The core muscles, including the rectus abdominis, obliques, and transverse abdominis, are responsible for maintaining proper body position and alignment in the water. A strong, stable core is essential for efficient swimming and injury prevention.

- Glutes and Legs: The gluteal muscles and leg muscles, particularly the quads and hamstrings, are responsible for generating propulsive force during kicking movements. Strong, powerful glutes and legs are essential for maintaining proper kicking technique and improving overall swimming speed.

## 3. Isometric Exercises for Swimmers

Here are some specific isometric exercises that can benefit swimmers:

- Isometric Shoulder External Rotation: Stand with your upper arm at your side and your elbow bent at a 90-degree angle, holding a resistance band or light dumbbell. Rotate your arm outward against resistance, holding for 30-60 seconds per side. This exercise targets the rotator cuff muscles.

- Isometric Pull-Up Hold: Hang from a pull-up bar with your palms facing away from you and your arms fully extended. Pull yourself up until your chin is above the bar, holding for 30-60 seconds. This exercise targets the lats and upper back muscles.

- Isometric Single-Arm Plank: Start in a plank position with your hands directly under your shoulders. Lift one arm off the ground, holding for 30-60 seconds per side. This exercise targets the core and shoulder stabilizers.

- Isometric Glute Bridge: Lie on your back with your knees bent and your feet flat on the ground. Lift your hips off the ground, squeezing your glutes and holding for 30-60 seconds. This exercise targets the glutes and hamstrings.

- Isometric Streamline Hold: Stand with your feet shoulder-width apart and your arms extended overhead in a streamline position, squeezing your shoulder blades together. Hold for 30-60 seconds, focusing on maintaining a tight, streamlined body position. This exercise targets the core, shoulders, and upper back.

## 4. Incorporating Isometric Exercises into Your Swim Training

To get the most benefit from isometric exercises, it's important to incorporate them into your swim training in a strategic way. Here are some tips:

- Perform isometric exercises 2-3 times per week, on non-swimming days or as part of your dryland training routine.
- Start with shorter hold times (10-20 seconds) and gradually progress to longer holds (30-60 seconds) as you build strength and endurance.

- Focus on maintaining proper form and alignment throughout each exercise, engaging the targeted muscle groups and avoiding compensatory movements.
- Pair isometric exercises with dynamic stretching and mobility work to maintain flexibility and range of motion.
- Listen to your body and adjust your training as needed to avoid overuse injuries or excessive fatigue.

## 5. Sample Isometric Workout for Swimmers

Here's a sample isometric workout that targets the key muscle groups for swimming:

1. Isometric Shoulder External Rotation: 3 sets of 45-second holds per arm
2. Isometric Pull-Up Hold: 3 sets of 60-second holds
3. Isometric Single-Arm Plank: 3 sets of 45-second holds per arm
4. Isometric Glute Bridge: 3 sets of 60-second holds
5. Isometric Streamline Hold: 3 sets of 60-second holds

Perform this workout 2-3 times per week, allowing for adequate rest and recovery between sessions.

## 6. Precautions and Considerations

While isometric exercises can be highly beneficial for swimmers, there are some precautions and considerations to keep in mind:

- If you have a history of shoulder injuries or pain, consult with a sports medicine professional before starting an isometric exercise program that targets the shoulders.

- If you experience pain or discomfort during any exercise, stop immediately and seek medical attention if necessary.
- Avoid holding your breath during isometric exercises, as this can cause a sudden spike in blood pressure. Focus on maintaining steady, controlled breathing throughout each hold.
- Don't neglect other aspects of your swim training, such as cardiovascular endurance, technique work, and flexibility. Isometric exercises should be one component of a well-rounded training program.

Incorporating isometric exercises into your swim training can help you build the strength, power, and stability you need to perform your best in the water. By targeting key muscle groups and maintaining proper form and technique, you can enhance your swimming efficiency and reduce your risk of injury.

So what are you waiting for? Dive into isometric training today and see the difference it can make in your swimming performance and overall health. Remember, consistency is key, and even small improvements can lead to big gains over time. Happy swimming!

# Tennis

Tennis is a dynamic, high-intensity sport that requires a combination of speed, agility, power, and endurance. Incorporating isometric exercises into your tennis training can help improve your performance on the court, increase your muscular strength and stability, and reduce your risk of injury.

Let's take a closer look at how isometric exercises can benefit tennis players and explore some specific exercises to incorporate into your training routine:

## 1. Benefits of Isometric Exercises for Tennis Players

Isometric exercises offer several key benefits for tennis players, including:

- Improved muscular strength: Tennis requires explosive movements and quick changes of direction, which demand high levels of muscular strength. Isometric exercises can help build the strength you need to generate powerful shots and maintain control on the court.

- Enhanced joint stability: Tennis involves repetitive, high-impact movements that can put stress on the joints, particularly the shoulders, elbows, and knees. Isometric exercises can help strengthen the muscles and connective tissues around these joints, improving stability and reducing the risk of injury.

- Increased core stability: A strong, stable core is essential for maintaining proper posture and balance during tennis strokes and movements. Isometric exercises that target the core, such as planks and side planks, can help improve your core stability and overall performance on the court.

- Greater muscular endurance: Tennis matches can last for several hours, requiring high levels of muscular endurance. Isometric exercises can help build the endurance you need to maintain proper form and technique throughout long rallies and matches.

## 2. Key Muscle Groups for Tennis Players

When incorporating isometric exercises into your tennis training, it's important to focus on the key muscle groups that are most important for tennis performance and injury prevention. These include:

- Shoulders: The shoulder muscles, particularly the rotator cuff and deltoids, are responsible for generating power and maintaining proper technique during serving and overhead shots. Strong, stable shoulders are essential for preventing overuse injuries like tennis elbow.

- Core: The core muscles, including the rectus abdominis, obliques, and transverse abdominis, are responsible for maintaining proper posture and balance during tennis strokes and movements. A strong, stable core is essential for generating power and maintaining control on the court.

- Legs: The leg muscles, particularly the quads, hamstrings, and calves, are responsible for generating explosive power and speed during tennis movements like sprinting, jumping, and lunging. Strong, powerful legs are essential for maintaining proper footwork and agility on the court.

- Forearms and Wrists: The forearm and wrist muscles are responsible for generating power and control during groundstrokes and volleys. Strong, stable forearms and wrists are essential for preventing overuse injuries like tennis elbow and wrist strains.

## 3. Isometric Exercises for Tennis Players

Here are some specific isometric exercises that can benefit tennis players:

- Isometric Wrist Extension: Stand with your forearm resting on a table and your hand hanging off the edge, holding a light dumbbell. Extend your wrist upward against resistance, holding for 30-60 seconds. This exercise targets the forearm extensors.

- Isometric Lateral Lunge: Stand with your feet wider than shoulder-width apart. Shift your weight to one leg, bending your knee and lowering your hips until your thigh is parallel to the ground. Hold for 30-60 seconds per side. This exercise targets the glutes, quads, and adductors.

- Isometric Rotator Cuff Hold: Stand with your elbow bent at a 90-degree angle and a resistance band anchored at shoulder height. Rotate your arm outward against resistance, holding for 30-60 seconds per side. This exercise targets the rotator cuff muscles.

- Isometric Single-Leg Calf Raise: Stand on one leg with your foot on the edge of a step or platform. Rise up onto your toes, holding for 30-60 seconds per leg. This exercise targets the calves.

- Isometric Plank with Arm Lift: Start in a plank position with your hands directly under your shoulders. Lift one arm off the ground, holding for 30-60 seconds per side. This exercise targets the core and shoulder stabilizers.

## 4. Incorporating Isometric Exercises into Your Tennis Training

To get the most benefit from isometric exercises, it's important to incorporate them into your tennis training in a strategic way. Here are some tips:

- Perform isometric exercises 2-3 times per week, on non-tennis days or as part of your strength and conditioning routine.
- Start with shorter hold times (10-20 seconds) and gradually progress to longer holds (30-60 seconds) as you build strength and endurance.
- Focus on maintaining proper form and alignment throughout each exercise, engaging the targeted muscle groups and avoiding compensatory movements.

- Pair isometric exercises with dynamic stretching and mobility work to maintain flexibility and range of motion.
- Listen to your body and adjust your training as needed to avoid overuse injuries or excessive fatigue.

## 5. Sample Isometric Workout for Tennis Players

Here's a sample isometric workout that targets the key muscle groups for tennis:

1. Isometric Wrist Extension: 3 sets of 45-second holds per arm
2. Isometric Lateral Lunge: 3 sets of 60-second holds per leg
3. Isometric Rotator Cuff Hold: 3 sets of 45-second holds per arm
4. Isometric Single-Leg Calf Raise: 3 sets of 60-second holds per leg
5. Isometric Plank with Arm Lift: 3 sets of 45-second holds per arm

Perform this workout 2-3 times per week, allowing for adequate rest and recovery between sessions.

## 6. Precautions and Considerations

While isometric exercises can be highly beneficial for tennis players, there are some precautions and considerations to keep in mind:

- If you have a history of joint injuries or pain, particularly in the shoulders, elbows, or knees, consult with a sports medicine professional before starting an isometric exercise program.

- If you experience pain or discomfort during any exercise, stop immediately and seek medical attention if necessary.
- Avoid holding your breath during isometric exercises, as this can cause a sudden spike in blood pressure. Focus on maintaining steady, controlled breathing throughout each hold.
- Don't neglect other aspects of your tennis training, such as cardiovascular endurance, footwork drills, and technique work. Isometric exercises should be one component of a well-rounded training program.

Incorporating isometric exercises into your tennis training can help you build the strength, stability, and endurance you need to perform your best on the court. By targeting key muscle groups and maintaining proper form and technique, you can enhance your tennis performance and reduce your risk of injury.

So what are you waiting for? Serve up some isometric training today and see the difference it can make in your tennis game and overall fitness. Remember, consistency is key, and even small improvements can lead to big gains over time. Happy hitting!

# Golf

In today's fast-paced, sedentary work environment, it's more important than ever to find ways to stay active and maintain good posture and muscle function throughout the day. Incorporating isometric exercises into your work routine can be a simple and effective way to boost your fitness, reduce stress, and improve your overall well-being.

Let's take a closer look at how you can integrate isometric exercises into your workday:

## 1. Desk-Friendly Isometric Exercises

Many isometric exercises can be performed right at your desk, without drawing too much attention or requiring any special equipment. Here are some examples:

- Isometric Glute Squeeze: While sitting in your chair, squeeze your glutes together as hard as you can, holding for 10-20 seconds at a time. Repeat for 3-5 sets throughout the day.

- Isometric Abdominal Brace: While sitting up straight in your chair, brace your abdominal muscles as if you were about to be punched in the gut. Hold for 10-20 seconds at a time, breathing normally throughout. Repeat for 3-5 sets throughout the day.

- Isometric Neck Retraction: While sitting up straight in your chair, tuck your chin down towards your chest and imagine pulling your head straight back. Hold for 10-20 seconds at a time, breathing normally throughout. Repeat for 3-5 sets throughout the day.

- Isometric Heel Raise: While sitting in your chair, press your toes into the ground and lift your heels as high as you can. Hold for 10-20 seconds at a time, feeling the contraction in your calf muscles. Repeat for 3-5 sets throughout the day.

## 2. Standing Isometric Exercises

If you have a standing desk or are able to take short breaks throughout the day to stand up and move around, there are even more isometric exercises you can incorporate into your work routine. Here are some examples:

- Isometric Wall Sit: Find a clear wall and lean back against it, sliding down until your knees are bent at a 90-degree angle. Hold this position for 30-60 seconds at a time, breathing normally throughout. Repeat for 2-3 sets throughout the day.

- Isometric Single-Leg Balance: Stand on one leg, keeping your other foot off the ground and your standing knee slightly bent. Hold this position for 30-60 seconds at a time, focusing on maintaining your balance and keeping your core engaged. Repeat on the other leg, and perform 2-3 sets throughout the day.

- Isometric Plank: Find a clear space on the floor and get into a plank position, with your forearms on the ground and your elbows directly under your shoulders. Hold this position for 30-60 seconds at a time, keeping your body in a straight line from head to heels. Repeat for 2-3 sets throughout the day.

- Isometric Lunge: Stand with one foot forward and one foot back, lowering your back knee towards the ground until both knees are bent at 90-degree angles. Hold this position for 30-60 seconds at a time, focusing on maintaining your balance and keeping your core engaged. Repeat on the other leg, and perform 2-3 sets throughout the day.

**3. Integrating Isometric Exercises into Your Work Routine**
To get the most benefit from isometric exercises at work, it's important to make them a regular part of your routine. Here are some tips for integrating isometric exercises into your workday:

- Set reminders: Use your phone, computer, or a sticky note to remind yourself to perform isometric exercises at regular intervals throughout the day, such as every hour or every 90 minutes.

- Start small: If you're new to isometric exercises, start with shorter hold times and fewer sets, and gradually build up as you get more comfortable and stronger.

- Be consistent: Try to perform isometric exercises at roughly the same times each day, so that they become a habit and a natural part of your work routine.

- Listen to your body: If you experience pain or discomfort during any exercise, stop immediately and seek medical attention if necessary. Isometric exercises should be challenging but not painful.

## 4. Benefits of Isometric Exercises at Work

Incorporating isometric exercises into your work routine can provide a range of benefits, including:

- Improved posture: Many isometric exercises, such as glute squeezes and abdominal braces, can help improve your posture by strengthening the muscles that support your spine and pelvis.

- Reduced risk of injury: By strengthening key muscle groups and improving your overall stability and balance, isometric exercises can help reduce your risk of workplace injuries, such as falls or strains.

- Increased energy and focus: Taking short breaks throughout the day to perform isometric exercises can help boost your energy levels and improve your mental focus, making you more productive and efficient at work.

- Reduced stress and tension: Isometric exercises can be a simple and effective way to relieve stress and tension throughout the workday, helping you feel more relaxed and centered.

Incorporating isometric exercises into your work routine can be a simple and effective way to stay active, healthy, and productive throughout the day. By taking short breaks to perform desk-friendly or standing isometric exercises, you can boost your fitness, reduce your risk of injury, and improve your overall well-being.

In today's modern work environment, many people spend long hours sitting at a desk, which can lead to poor posture, muscle weakness, and various health issues. Incorporating isometric exercises into your workday can help combat these problems, improve your overall well-being, and boost your productivity. Let's explore how you can effectively integrate isometric exercises into your work routine.

## 1. Understanding the Benefits of Isometric Exercises at Work

Performing isometric exercises at work offers several key advantages:

a. Convenience: Isometric exercises can be done at your desk or workstation without requiring any special equipment or space.

b. Time-efficient: These exercises can be completed in short bursts throughout the day, making them easy to fit into even the busiest schedules.

c. Discreet: Many isometric exercises are subtle and can be performed without drawing attention to yourself, making them ideal for the workplace.

d. Posture improvement: Isometric exercises can help strengthen the muscles responsible for maintaining good posture, reducing the risk of back pain and other posture-related issues.

e. Stress relief: Engaging in isometric exercises can provide a mental break and help alleviate stress and tension that often accompany work.

**2. Isometric Exercises for the Workplace**
Here are some effective isometric exercises you can perform at work:

a. Desk plank: Place your hands on the edge of your desk, shoulder-width apart. Walk your feet back until your body forms a straight line from head to heels. Hold this position for 30-60 seconds, engaging your core and maintaining proper alignment.

b. Chair squats: Stand in front of your chair with your feet shoulder-width apart. Lower yourself down as if you were going to sit, but stop just before your buttocks touch the chair. Hold this position for 30-60 seconds, keeping your back straight and your core engaged.

c. Seated leg raises: While seated, extend one leg out in front of you, keeping it as straight as possible. Hold for 10-15 seconds, then lower it back down. Repeat with the other leg. Aim for 3-5 sets on each leg.

d. Isometric push-ups: Place your hands on the edge of your desk, slightly wider than shoulder-width apart. Lower your chest towards the desk, keeping your body in a straight line. Hold this position for 30-60 seconds, focusing on maintaining proper form.

e. Wall sits: Find a clear wall space and lean back against it, lowering yourself down until your thighs are parallel to the ground. Hold this position for 30-60 seconds, keeping your back pressed against the wall and your core engaged.

## 3. Implementing Isometric Exercises into Your Work Routine

To make isometric exercises a consistent part of your workday, try these tips:

a. Set reminders: Use your phone, computer, or a sticky note to remind yourself to perform isometric exercises at regular intervals throughout the day.

b. Start small: Begin with shorter hold times and fewer sets, gradually increasing the duration and intensity as you build strength and endurance.

c. Pair exercises with tasks: Associate specific isometric exercises with certain work tasks, such as performing desk planks while waiting for a document to print or doing chair squats while on a conference call.

d. Involve coworkers: Encourage your colleagues to join you in performing isometric exercises, creating a supportive and accountable work environment.

e. Listen to your body: If you experience pain or discomfort during any exercise, stop immediately and consult with a healthcare professional if necessary.

## 4. Precautions and Considerations

While isometric exercises are generally safe and beneficial, there are a few precautions to keep in mind:

a. Breathing: Avoid holding your breath during isometric exercises, as this can cause a sudden spike in blood pressure. Focus on maintaining steady, controlled breathing throughout each exercise.

b. Pre-existing conditions: If you have a history of high blood pressure, heart disease, or other cardiovascular concerns, consult with your doctor before starting an isometric exercise routine.

c. Proper form: Maintain proper alignment and technique during each exercise to prevent strain or injury. If you're unsure about how to perform an exercise correctly, seek guidance from a fitness professional.

d. Workstation ergonomics: Ensure that your workstation is set up ergonomically to support good posture and reduce the risk of strain or injury during isometric exercises.

## 5. Progressing and Varying Your Isometric Exercises

As you become more comfortable with isometric exercises, consider these ways to progress and vary your routine:

a. Increase hold times: Gradually increase the duration of each isometric hold, working up to 60-90 seconds per exercise.

b. Add resistance: Incorporate resistance bands or small weights to increase the challenge of certain exercises, such as seated leg raises or isometric push-ups.

c. Try new exercises: Expand your repertoire of isometric exercises to target different muscle groups and keep your routine engaging.

d. Combine with dynamic movements: Integrate isometric holds with dynamic stretches or movements to create a more comprehensive workday wellness routine.

Incorporating isometric exercises into your work routine is a simple, effective way to improve your physical health, mental well-being, and overall productivity. By making these exercises a consistent part of your workday, you can combat the negative effects of prolonged sitting, reduce stress, and maintain a stronger, more resilient body.

Remember, the key to success with isometric exercises at work is consistency and progression. Start small, set reminders, and gradually build upon your routine over time. With dedication and regular practice, you'll be amazed at the positive impact these simple exercises can have on your work life and overall health.

Traveling can disrupt your normal fitness routine, making it challenging to maintain your strength and overall well-being. Whether you're on a business trip or a family vacation, incorporating isometric exercises into your travel routine can help you stay active, reduce stress, and prevent muscle atrophy. Let's explore how you can effectively perform isometric exercises while on the go.

**1. Benefits of Isometric Exercises While Traveling**

Engaging in isometric exercises while traveling offers several key advantages:

a. No equipment necessary: Isometric exercises rely on your body's own resistance, eliminating the need for bulky equipment or weights.

b. Space-efficient: These exercises can be performed in small spaces, such as hotel rooms, airport lounges, or even airplane seats.

c. Time-saving: Isometric exercises can be completed in short sessions throughout the day, making them easy to fit into a busy travel schedule.

d. Stress relief: Traveling can be stressful, and isometric exercises can help alleviate tension, promote relaxation, and improve overall mood.

e. Muscle maintenance: Regularly performing isometric exercises while traveling can help prevent muscle loss and maintain your strength until you can resume your normal fitness routine.

## 2. Isometric Exercises for Travel

Here are some effective isometric exercises you can perform while traveling:

a. Suitcase deadlifts: Place your suitcase on the ground in front of you. Hinge at your hips, keeping your back straight, and grab the suitcase handles. Squeeze your glutes and engage your core as you lift the suitcase a few inches off the ground. Hold for 10-15 seconds, then lower it back down. Repeat for 3-5 sets.

b. Wall push-ups: Find a clear wall space and place your hands on the wall, slightly wider than shoulder-width apart. Lower your chest towards the wall, keeping your body in a straight line. Hold this position for 30-60 seconds, focusing on maintaining proper form.

c. Seated ab contractions: While seated in a chair or airplane seat, sit up tall and engage your abdominal muscles, pulling your belly button towards your spine. Hold this contraction for 10-15 seconds, then release. Repeat for 3-5 sets.

d. Isometric squats: Stand with your feet shoulder-width apart and your back against a wall. Lower yourself down into a squat position, as if you were sitting back into a chair. Hold this position for 30-60 seconds, keeping your core engaged and your back pressed against the wall.

e. Luggage rows: Place your suitcase on a bed or elevated surface. Hinge at your hips, keeping your back straight, and grab the suitcase handles. Pull the suitcase towards your chest, squeezing your shoulder blades together. Hold this position for 10-15 seconds, then lower the suitcase back down. Repeat for 3-5 sets.

## 3. Incorporating Isometric Exercises into Your Travel Routine

To make isometric exercises a consistent part of your travel routine, try these tips:

a. Schedule exercise breaks: Set aside specific times throughout the day to perform isometric exercises, such as first thing in the morning or during layovers.

b. Utilize downtime: Take advantage of idle time, such as waiting in line or sitting on a plane, to perform seated or standing isometric exercises discreetly.

c. Create a travel-friendly workout plan: Before your trip, design a simple isometric exercise routine that you can easily follow while on the go.

d. Stay accountable: Use a travel journal or fitness app to track your isometric exercise sessions and maintain motivation.

e. Adapt to your environment: Be creative and look for opportunities to perform isometric exercises using your surroundings, such as luggage, hotel furniture, or even your own body weight.

## 4. Precautions and Considerations

When performing isometric exercises while traveling, keep these precautions in mind:

a. Breathing: Maintain steady, controlled breathing throughout each exercise to avoid sudden spikes in blood pressure.

b. Space awareness: Be mindful of your surroundings and ensure that you have enough space to perform each exercise safely and without disturbing others.

c. Listen to your body: If you experience pain or discomfort during any exercise, stop immediately and consult with a healthcare professional if necessary.

d. Hydration: Stay well-hydrated throughout your travels to support your overall health and exercise performance.

5. Progressing and Varying Your Travel Isometric Exercises
To keep your travel isometric routine challenging and engaging, consider these ways to progress and vary your exercises:

a. Increase hold times: Gradually increase the duration of each isometric hold, working up to 60-90 seconds per exercise.

b. Incorporate multiple planes of motion: Include isometric exercises that target different planes of motion, such as front-to-back, side-to-side, and rotational movements.

c. Combine with dynamic stretches: Integrate isometric holds with dynamic stretches to create a more comprehensive travel fitness routine that addresses both strength and flexibility.

d. Explore local fitness opportunities: Look for chances to engage in isometric exercises at your destination, such as participating in a yoga class or trying a local park workout.

Incorporating isometric exercises into your travel routine is an effective way to maintain your strength, reduce stress, and promote overall well-being while on the go. By making these exercises a consistent part of your travel experience, you can ensure that your fitness goals don't take a backseat during your adventures.

Remember, the key to success with travel isometric exercises is adaptability and consistency. Embrace the challenges of your new environment, find creative ways to incorporate isometric exercises into your daily routine, and stay committed to your fitness goals. With a little planning and dedication, you can return from your travels feeling stronger, more resilient, and ready to tackle whatever comes your way.

# Isometric Exercises for Active Recovery Days

Active recovery days are an essential component of any well-rounded fitness routine. These days are designed to help your body recover from intense workouts while still maintaining a level of physical activity. Incorporating isometric exercises into your active recovery days can offer numerous benefits, promoting muscle recovery, reducing soreness, and improving overall flexibility and range of motion. Let's dive deeper into how isometric exercises can enhance your active recovery sessions.

## 1. Understanding Active Recovery

Active recovery involves engaging in low-intensity exercises or activities that stimulate blood flow and promote muscle recovery without adding significant stress to the body. The main goals of active recovery are to:

a. Reduce muscle soreness and stiffness
b. Flush out metabolic waste products, such as lactic acid
c. Improve circulation and nutrient delivery to muscles
d. Maintain flexibility and range of motion
e. Promote relaxation and mental well-being

2. Benefits of Isometric Exercises for Active Recovery
Incorporating isometric exercises into your active recovery days offers several key advantages:

a. Low-impact: Isometric exercises place minimal stress on the joints and connective tissues, making them ideal for recovery sessions when the body needs a break from high-impact activities.

b. Targeted muscle activation: Isometric exercises allow you to focus on specific muscle groups, promoting blood flow and aiding in the recovery process.

c. Versatility: These exercises can be performed anywhere, without the need for equipment, making them convenient for recovery sessions at home or on the go.

d. Improved mind-muscle connection: Isometric exercises require a strong focus on muscle contraction and body awareness, enhancing the mind-muscle connection and promoting relaxation.

e. Flexibility and range of motion: Holding isometric stretches can help improve flexibility and range of motion, which are crucial for maintaining healthy, resilient muscles.

**3. Isometric Exercises for Active Recovery Sessions**
Here are some effective isometric exercises to include in your active recovery days:

a. Isometric chest stretch: Stand in a doorway with your arms bent at 90-degree angles, forearms resting on the door frame. Step forward, feeling a stretch across your chest. Hold for 30-60 seconds, then release.

b. Isometric quadriceps hold: Lie on your stomach with a rolled-up towel under your right ankle. Contract your right quadriceps muscle, pressing your ankle into the towel. Hold for 10-15 seconds, then release. Repeat on the left leg.

c. Isometric shoulder external rotation: Stand with your right side next to a wall, upper arm pressed against your body, and elbow bent at a 90-degree angle. Press the back of your hand into the wall, contracting your shoulder external rotators. Hold for 10-15 seconds, then release. Repeat on the left side.

d. Isometric glute bridge hold: Lie on your back with your knees bent and feet flat on the floor. Lift your hips off the ground, squeezing your glutes. Hold this position for 30-60 seconds, focusing on maintaining a strong glute contraction.

e. Isometric calf stretch: Stand facing a wall, placing your hands on the wall for support. Step back with your right leg, keeping your heel on the ground. Lean forward, feeling a stretch in your right calf. Hold for 30-60 seconds, then release. Repeat on the left leg.

**4. Incorporating Isometric Exercises into Your Active Recovery Routine**
To effectively integrate isometric exercises into your active recovery days, consider these tips:

a. Timing: Perform isometric exercises on days following intense workouts or on designated rest days.

b. Duration: Aim for 10-20 minutes of total isometric exercise time during each active recovery session.

c. Progression: Gradually increase the hold times for each isometric exercise as your body adapts and becomes more comfortable with the movements.

d. Breathing: Focus on deep, controlled breathing throughout each isometric hold to promote relaxation and oxygenation of the muscles.

e. Complementary activities: Combine isometric exercises with other low-intensity activities, such as walking, swimming, or yoga, to create a well-rounded active recovery routine.

## 5. Precautions and Considerations

When incorporating isometric exercises into your active recovery days, keep these precautions in mind:

a. Proper form: Maintain proper alignment and technique during each isometric hold to prevent undue strain on the muscles or joints.

b. Pain awareness: If you experience sharp pain or discomfort during any isometric exercise, stop immediately and reassess your form or consult with a healthcare professional.

c. Hydration: Stay well-hydrated before, during, and after your active recovery sessions to support muscle recovery and overall health.

d. Individualization: Adjust your isometric exercises and hold times based on your fitness level, recovery needs, and personal preferences.

## 6. Sample Isometric Active Recovery Routine

Here's an example of a 15-minute isometric active recovery routine:

a. Isometric chest stretch: 2 sets of 30-second holds
b. Isometric quadriceps hold: 2 sets of 15-second holds per leg
c. Isometric shoulder external rotation: 2 sets of 15-second holds per arm
d. Isometric glute bridge hold: 2 sets of 45-second holds
e. Isometric calf stretch: 2 sets of 30-second holds per leg

Remember to focus on deep breathing and muscle relaxation throughout the routine.

Incorporating isometric exercises into your active recovery days is a simple and effective way to promote muscle recovery, reduce soreness, and maintain flexibility. By dedicating time to these low-impact exercises, you can support your body's natural healing processes and enhance your overall fitness progress.

As with any new exercise routine, listen to your body and adjust your isometric active recovery plan as needed. Consistency and patience are key – over time, you'll likely notice improvements in your muscle recovery, flexibility, and overall well-being.

Embrace the power of isometric exercises on your active recovery days, and watch as your body becomes more resilient, adaptable, and ready to tackle your next workout with renewed energy and strength.

Combating Sedentary Behavior with Isometric Exercises uding obesity, cardiovascular disease, and musculoskeletal problems. Incorporating isometric exercises into your daily routine can help combat the negative effects of sedentary behavior, promoting better health and overall well-being. Let's explore how isometric exercises can be a powerful tool in fighting sedentary lifestyle habits.

## 1. The Risks of Sedentary Behavior

Sedentary behavior refers to any waking activity characterized by low energy expenditure and a sitting, reclining, or lying posture. Prolonged sedentary time can contribute to various health concerns, such as:

a. Obesity and metabolic disorders
b. Cardiovascular disease
c. Type 2 diabetes
d. Certain types of cancer
e. Musculoskeletal problems, such as back pain and poor posture
f. Mental health issues, including depression and anxiety

## 2. How Isometric Exercises Can Help Combat Sedentary Behavior

Incorporating isometric exercises into your daily routine can help counteract the negative effects of sedentary behavior in several ways:

a. Increased muscle activation: Isometric exercises involve sustained muscle contractions, which can help activate and strengthen muscles that may become weak or underutilized due to prolonged sitting.

b. Improved circulation: By contracting muscles during isometric exercises, you can stimulate blood flow and improve circulation throughout the body, reducing the risk of blood clots and other cardiovascular issues associated with prolonged sitting.

c. Enhanced postural awareness: Performing isometric exercises requires focus on proper alignment and body positioning, which can translate into improved posture during daily activities, reducing the risk of musculoskeletal problems.

d. Increased energy expenditure: While isometric exercises may not burn as many calories as dynamic movements, they still contribute to overall energy expenditure, helping to combat the effects of prolonged inactivity.

e. Mental breaks and stress relief: Engaging in isometric exercises throughout the day can provide mental breaks from sedentary tasks, reducing stress and promoting a more positive mindset.

**3. Isometric Exercises for Combating Sedentary Behavior**
Here are some simple yet effective isometric exercises that you can incorporate into your daily routine to combat sedentary behavior:

a. Seated leg extensions: While sitting, extend one leg out in front of you, contracting your quadriceps muscle. Hold for 10-15 seconds, then release. Repeat on the opposite leg.

b. Desk plank holds: Place your hands on the edge of your desk, shoulder-width apart. Walk your feet back until your body forms a straight line from head to heels. Hold this position for 30-60 seconds, engaging your core and maintaining proper alignment.

c. Isometric glute squeezes: While sitting, contract your glute muscles, squeezing them as tightly as possible. Hold for 10-15 seconds, then release. Repeat for 3-5 sets throughout the day.

d. Wall push-ups: Stand facing a wall, placing your hands on the wall at shoulder height. Lean in, bending your elbows, and press your body weight against the wall. Hold for 30-60 seconds, maintaining a straight line from head to heels.

e. Seated abdominal contractions: While sitting up tall, contract your abdominal muscles, pulling your belly button towards your spine. Hold for 10-15 seconds, then release. Repeat for 3-5 sets.

**4. Incorporating Isometric Exercises into Your Daily Routine**

To effectively combat sedentary behavior, make isometric exercises a consistent part of your daily routine:

a. Set reminders: Use your phone, computer, or a sticky note to remind yourself to perform isometric exercises at regular intervals throughout the day, such as every hour.

b. Create an exercise-friendly workspace: Ensure that your workspace allows for easy incorporation of isometric exercises, such as having enough room to perform desk planks or wall push-ups.

c. Make it a habit: Pair isometric exercises with specific daily tasks or routines, such as performing seated leg extensions while on phone calls or doing isometric glute squeezes during commercial breaks.

d. Involve others: Encourage coworkers, family members, or friends to join you in incorporating isometric exercises into their daily routines, creating a supportive and accountable environment.

## 5. Precautions and Considerations

When using isometric exercises to combat sedentary behavior, keep these precautions in mind:

a. Proper form: Maintain proper alignment and technique during each exercise to prevent strain or injury.

b. Breathing: Avoid holding your breath during isometric exercises, as this can cause a sudden spike in blood pressure. Focus on maintaining steady, controlled breathing throughout each contraction.

c. Gradual progression: Begin with shorter hold times and fewer sets, gradually increasing the duration and frequency as your body adapts to the exercises.

d. Listening to your body: If you experience pain or discomfort during any isometric exercise, stop immediately and reassess your form or consult with a healthcare professional.

6. Complementary Strategies to Combat Sedentary Behavior
While isometric exercises can be a powerful tool in fighting sedentary behavior, they should be combined with other strategies for optimal results:

a. Take regular breaks: Stand up and move around every 30-60 minutes, even if just for a few minutes, to promote circulation and reduce prolonged sitting.

b. Incorporate dynamic movements: Engage in activities that involve dynamic movements, such as walking, stretching, or light calisthenics, to complement your isometric exercises and promote overall physical activity.

c. Prioritize ergonomics: Ensure that your workspace is set up ergonomically, with proper chair height, computer monitor positioning, and lumbar support to reduce the risk of musculoskeletal issues.

d. Maintain a balanced lifestyle: Alongside isometric exercises, prioritize other healthy lifestyle habits, such as regular exercise, a balanced diet, and adequate sleep, to combat the overall effects of sedentary behavior.

Incorporating isometric exercises into your daily routine is a simple and effective way to combat the negative effects of sedentary behavior. By consistently engaging in these exercises and combining them with other strategies to reduce prolonged sitting, you can promote better health, improve your posture, and enhance your overall well-being.

Remember, small changes can lead to significant improvements over time. Start by incorporating a few isometric exercises into your day and gradually build upon your routine as you become more comfortable with the movements. With dedication and consistency, you'll be well on your way to combating sedentary behavior and enjoying the numerous benefits of a more active lifestyle.

Proper nutrition plays a crucial role in supporting your isometric exercise routine and optimizing your results. By providing your body with the right nutrients, you can enhance your performance, promote muscle recovery, and reduce the risk of injury. Let's dive into the essential aspects of nutrition for isometric exercise success.

**1. The Role of Nutrition in Isometric Exercise**
Nutrition is a key factor in any fitness program, and isometric exercises are no exception. Proper nutrition can support your isometric training in several ways:

a. Energy provision: Consuming a balanced diet with adequate carbohydrates, fats, and proteins ensures that your body has the energy needed to perform isometric exercises effectively.

b. Muscle recovery: Eating nutrient-dense foods, particularly those rich in protein, helps repair and rebuild muscle tissue after isometric training sessions.

c. Injury prevention: Adequate nutrition supports the health and resilience of your muscles, tendons, and ligaments, reducing the risk of injury during isometric exercises.

d. Overall health: A well-balanced diet promotes overall health and well-being, enabling you to perform at your best during isometric training and in daily life.

## 2. Macronutrients for Isometric Exercise

To fuel your body for isometric exercise success, focus on consuming a balance of the three primary macronutrients:

a. Carbohydrates: Carbohydrates are the body's primary energy source. Consume complex carbohydrates, such as whole grains, fruits, and vegetables, to provide sustained energy for your isometric workouts.

b. Proteins: Proteins are essential for muscle repair and growth. Include lean protein sources, such as chicken, fish, tofu, and legumes, in your diet to support muscle recovery after isometric training.

c. Fats: Healthy fats, such as those found in avocados, nuts, seeds, and olive oil, are important for hormone production, nutrient absorption, and overall health. Incorporate moderate amounts of healthy fats into your diet to support your isometric exercise routine.

## 3. Pre and Post-Workout Nutrition

What you eat before and after your isometric training sessions can significantly impact your performance and recovery. Here are some guidelines for pre and post-workout nutrition:

a. Pre-workout: Consume a balanced meal containing complex carbohydrates and lean protein 2-3 hours before your isometric workout. This will provide sustained energy and support muscle function during your training session.

b. Post-workout: After your isometric workout, consume a meal or snack containing both protein and carbohydrates within 30-60 minutes. This will help replenish energy stores, promote muscle recovery, and reduce muscle soreness.

## 4. Hydration for Isometric Exercise

Proper hydration is crucial for optimal performance and recovery during isometric training. Follow these tips to stay well-hydrated:

a. Drink water consistently throughout the day, aiming for at least 8 glasses (64 ounces) of water per day.

b. Consume fluids before, during, and after your isometric workouts to replace fluids lost through sweat and maintain optimal hydration levels.

c. If you're exercising intensely or in hot conditions, consider using an electrolyte replacement drink to replenish lost minerals.

## 5. Nutrient-Dense Foods for Isometric Exercise

To support your isometric training, focus on incorporating a variety of nutrient-dense foods into your diet:

a. Fruits and vegetables: Aim to consume a rainbow of fruits and vegetables to ensure a wide range of vitamins, minerals, and antioxidants that support overall health and recovery.

b. Whole grains: Choose whole grain options, such as brown rice, quinoa, and whole wheat bread, for sustained energy and fiber.

c. Lean proteins: Include lean protein sources, such as chicken, fish, tofu, and legumes, to support muscle repair and growth.

d. Healthy fats: Incorporate healthy fat sources, such as avocados, nuts, seeds, and olive oil, to support hormone production and overall health.

## 6. Supplements for Isometric Exercise

While a well-balanced diet should be the foundation of your nutrition plan, certain supplements may be beneficial for supporting your isometric training:

a. Protein powder: A high-quality protein powder can be a convenient way to increase your protein intake and support muscle recovery after isometric workouts.

b. Creatine: Creatine is a naturally occurring compound that can help improve strength and muscle mass. It may be particularly beneficial for those engaging in high-intensity isometric training.

c. Omega-3 fatty acids: Omega-3 supplements, such as fish oil, can help reduce inflammation and support overall health.

Before starting any supplement regimen, consult with a healthcare professional to ensure safety and appropriateness for your individual needs.

## 7. Meal Planning and Preparation

To ensure that you're consistently fueling your body for isometric exercise success, consider implementing meal planning and preparation strategies:

a. Plan your meals and snacks in advance, focusing on incorporating a balance of macronutrients and nutrient-dense foods.

b. Prepare meals and snacks ahead of time to ensure that you always have healthy options readily available, even on busy days.

c. Keep healthy snacks, such as fresh fruits, vegetables, and nuts, on hand for quick and easy fueling before or after your isometric workouts.

d. Consider using a food tracking app or journal to monitor your nutrient intake and ensure that you're meeting your dietary needs.

By prioritizing proper nutrition and fueling your body with the right nutrients, you can optimize your performance, recovery, and results from your isometric exercise routine. Remember, consistency is key – aim to make healthy eating a long-term lifestyle habit rather than a short-term fix.

As you progress in your isometric training, pay attention to how your body responds to different foods and adjust your nutrition plan accordingly. With dedication and a balanced approach to nutrition, you'll be well on your way to achieving your isometric exercise goals and enjoying the numerous benefits of a healthy, active lifestyle.

Hydration is a crucial aspect of overall health and well-being, playing a vital role in various bodily functions and processes. When it comes to isometric exercise, proper hydration becomes even more critical, as it directly impacts performance, recovery, and the body's ability to adapt to the demands of training. Let's take an in-depth look at the importance of hydration and how it relates to isometric exercise.

## 1. The Role of Water in the Body

Water is essential for life, making up a significant portion of the human body. It plays a key role in numerous bodily functions, including:

a. Nutrient transport: Water helps dissolve and transport nutrients, such as vitamins and minerals, throughout the body, ensuring that cells receive the necessary compounds for optimal function.

b. Waste removal: Water aids in the removal of metabolic waste products, such as urea and carbon dioxide, through urine and sweat.

c. Temperature regulation: Through sweating and evaporation, water helps regulate body temperature, preventing overheating during physical activity.

d. Joint lubrication: Water is a key component of synovial fluid, which lubricates and cushions joints, reducing friction and supporting smooth movement.

e. Cellular function: Water is essential for maintaining the structure and function of cells, as it is involved in various cellular processes, such as nutrient uptake and enzymatic reactions.

## 2. Dehydration and Its Effects on Isometric Exercise Performance

Dehydration occurs when the body loses more fluids than it takes in, leading to an imbalance in water and electrolytes. Even mild dehydration can have significant effects on isometric exercise performance:

a. Reduced muscle strength: Dehydration can lead to decreased muscle strength and power output, making it more difficult to maintain isometric contractions and perform at a high level.

b. Increased fatigue: When dehydrated, the body has to work harder to maintain normal functions, leading to increased fatigue and reduced endurance during isometric exercises.

c. Impaired cognitive function: Dehydration can negatively impact cognitive function, including focus, decision-making, and reaction time, which can hinder performance during isometric training sessions.

d. Increased risk of injury: Dehydration can contribute to muscle cramps, strains, and other injuries, as the muscles and connective tissues are more susceptible to damage when the body is not adequately hydrated.

## 3. Hydration and Muscle Recovery

Proper hydration is essential for optimal muscle recovery after isometric training sessions:

a. Nutrient delivery: Water helps transport nutrients, such as amino acids and glucose, to the muscles, supporting repair and rebuilding processes.

b. Waste removal: Adequate hydration aids in the removal of metabolic waste products, such as lactic acid, from the muscles, reducing soreness and promoting faster recovery.

c. Protein synthesis: Hydration plays a role in protein synthesis, the process by which the body builds new muscle tissue. Dehydration can impair this process, slowing down muscle recovery and growth.

## 4. Electrolyte Balance and Isometric Exercise

In addition to water, electrolytes are crucial for maintaining optimal hydration and supporting isometric exercise performance:

a. Sodium: Sodium helps regulate fluid balance in the body, and it is lost through sweat during exercise. Adequate sodium intake is necessary to maintain proper hydration and prevent hyponatremia (low blood sodium levels).

b. Potassium: Potassium is essential for muscle and nerve function, and it is also lost through sweat. Maintaining proper potassium levels can help prevent muscle cramps and support optimal muscle contraction during isometric exercises.

c. Magnesium: Magnesium plays a role in energy production, muscle function, and nervous system regulation. Adequate magnesium intake can support muscle recovery and reduce the risk of muscle cramps and spasms.

## 5. Hydration Strategies for Isometric Exercise

To ensure optimal hydration for isometric exercise, consider the following strategies:

a. Pre-exercise hydration: Drink 16-20 ounces of water 2-3 hours before your isometric training session to ensure adequate hydration at the start of your workout.

b. During exercise: Drink 4-8 ounces of water every 15-20 minutes during your isometric training session to replace fluids lost through sweat and maintain optimal hydration levels.

c. Post-exercise hydration: After your isometric workout, drink 16-24 ounces of water for every pound of body weight lost during the session to replenish fluids and support recovery.

d. Electrolyte replacement: If you're exercising intensely or in hot conditions, consider using an electrolyte replacement drink or consuming foods rich in electrolytes, such as bananas, spinach, and avocados, to maintain proper electrolyte balance.

## 6. Monitoring Hydration Status

To ensure that you're adequately hydrated, monitor your hydration status using these simple methods:

a. Urine color: Clear or light yellow urine indicates adequate hydration, while dark yellow or amber-colored urine suggests dehydration.

b. Thirst: Thirst is a signal that your body needs fluids. If you feel thirsty, drink water or an electrolyte replacement drink to rehydrate.

c. Body weight: Weighing yourself before and after exercise can help you determine how much fluid you've lost through sweat. Aim to replace each pound of body weight lost with 16-24 ounces of fluids.

## 7. Hydration and Overall Health

In addition to its importance for isometric exercise performance and recovery, proper hydration is crucial for overall health and well-being:

a. Digestive health: Water aids in the digestion and absorption of nutrients, and it helps prevent constipation by keeping the digestive tract lubricated.

b. Skin health: Adequate hydration helps maintain skin elasticity and moisture, reducing the appearance of fine lines and wrinkles and promoting a healthy, glowing complexion.

c. Kidney function: Water is essential for kidney function, as it helps flush out toxins and waste products, preventing the formation of kidney stones and other renal issues.

d. Immune function: Proper hydration supports immune function by aiding in the production and circulation of lymph, a fluid that contains infection-fighting white blood cells.

By prioritizing hydration and making it a key component of your isometric exercise routine and overall lifestyle, you can optimize your performance, recovery, and health. Remember to drink water consistently throughout the day, and pay attention to your body's thirst signals to ensure that you're meeting your hydration needs.

As you progress in your isometric training, experiment with different hydration strategies and find what works best for you. With dedication and a proactive approach to hydration, you'll be well on your way to achieving your isometric exercise goals and enjoying the numerous benefits of a well-hydrated, healthy body.

## Stretching and Mobility Work

Stretching and mobility work are essential components of optimizing recovery and maximizing the results of your isometric training program. These practices help improve flexibility, reduce muscle tension, and enhance overall range of motion, all of which contribute to better performance and reduced risk of injury. Let's take an in-depth look at the benefits of stretching and mobility work and how to incorporate them into your recovery routine.

### 1. The Benefits of Stretching and Mobility Work

Regular stretching and mobility work offer numerous benefits for recovery and overall fitness:

a. Improved flexibility: Stretching helps lengthen muscles and improve overall flexibility, which can enhance performance and reduce the risk of injury during isometric exercises.

b. Reduced muscle tension: Stretching and mobility work help reduce muscle tension and tightness, which can accumulate during isometric training and contribute to discomfort and impaired recovery.

c. Increased range of motion: By improving flexibility and reducing muscle tension, stretching and mobility work can help increase overall range of motion, allowing for more efficient and effective movement patterns during isometric exercises.

d. Enhanced circulation: Stretching and mobility work can help increase blood flow and circulation to the muscles, which supports the delivery of oxygen and nutrients necessary for recovery and repair.

e. Improved posture: Regular stretching and mobility work can help improve posture by addressing muscle imbalances and promoting proper alignment, which can reduce the risk of injury and enhance overall well-being.

## 2. Types of Stretching

There are several types of stretching that can be incorporated into your recovery routine:

a. Static stretching: This involves holding a stretch in a stationary position for a period of time, typically 15-30 seconds. Static stretching is best performed after exercise when the muscles are warm and more pliable.

b. Dynamic stretching: This involves moving through a range of motion in a controlled manner, often mimicking the movements of the activity or exercise you are about to perform. Dynamic stretching is best performed before exercise as a part of a warm-up routine.

c. Proprioceptive Neuromuscular Facilitation (PNF) stretching: This advanced form of stretching involves alternating between muscle contractions and relaxation to achieve a deeper stretch. PNF stretching is best performed with the guidance of a trained professional.

## 3. Mobility Work

Mobility work involves exercises and drills designed to improve overall range of motion and movement quality:

a. Joint mobilization: This involves targeting specific joints, such as the hips, shoulders, and ankles, with exercises that promote mobility and reduce restriction.

b. Soft tissue work: This involves using tools such as foam rollers, massage balls, and stick massagers to address muscle tension and trigger points, promoting relaxation and improved mobility.

c. Dynamic movement drills: These involve moving through a range of motion in a functional, multi-joint manner to improve overall movement quality and coordination.

## 4. Incorporating Stretching and Mobility Work into Your Recovery Routine

To optimize recovery and maximize the benefits of stretching and mobility work, consider the following guidelines:

a. Stretch after exercise: Perform static stretching after your isometric training sessions when your muscles are warm and more receptive to stretching. Hold each stretch for 15-30 seconds and repeat 2-4 times for each muscle group.

b. Incorporate dynamic stretching into your warm-up: Before your isometric training sessions, perform dynamic stretching to prepare your body for the demands of exercise. Focus on movements that mimic the exercises you will be performing.

c. Perform mobility work regularly: Incorporate mobility work into your routine on a daily basis, even on non-training days. Focus on targeting areas of restriction and improving overall movement quality.

d. Listen to your body: Stretching and mobility work should never be painful. Listen to your body and respect your current level of flexibility and mobility, gradually progressing over time.

## 5. Sample Stretching and Mobility Routine

Here is a sample stretching and mobility routine that can be incorporated into your recovery program:

a. Static Stretches (perform after isometric training):
- Hamstring stretch: 30 seconds each leg
- Quadriceps stretch: 30 seconds each leg
- Chest stretch: 30 seconds each arm
- Triceps stretch: 30 seconds each arm
- Shoulder stretch: 30 seconds each arm

b. Dynamic Stretches (perform before isometric training):
- Leg swings: 10 repetitions each leg
- Arm circles: 10 repetitions each direction
- Lunges with trunk rotation: 10 repetitions each side
- High knees: 30 seconds
- Butt kicks: 30 seconds

c. Mobility Work (perform daily):
- Foam rolling: 5-10 minutes targeting major muscle groups

- Hip mobility drills: 5-10 repetitions each exercise
- Shoulder mobility drills: 5-10 repetitions each exercise
- Ankle mobility drills: 5-10 repetitions each exercise

Remember to adapt this routine to your individual needs and goals, and to gradually progress over time to avoid injury and promote optimal recovery.

## 6. Precautions and Considerations

While stretching and mobility work are generally safe and beneficial, there are a few precautions to keep in mind:

a. Avoid overstretching: Stretching should never be painful. Overstretching can lead to muscle strain and impaired recovery. Focus on gentle, gradual lengthening of the muscles.

b. Don't stretch cold muscles: Always perform stretching after exercise or after a gentle warm-up to avoid injury. Cold muscles are more susceptible to strain and tear.

c. Be mindful of existing injuries: If you have an existing injury or condition, consult with a healthcare professional before starting a new stretching or mobility routine to ensure safety and appropriateness.

d. Maintain proper form: Proper form and technique are essential for effective stretching and mobility work. If you are unsure about how to perform a specific exercise or stretch, seek guidance from a qualified fitness professional.

By incorporating regular stretching and mobility work into your recovery routine, you can improve flexibility, reduce muscle tension, enhance range of motion, and support overall recovery and performance. Remember to listen to your body, start slowly, and gradually progress over time to avoid injury and maximize the benefits of these practices.

As you continue on your isometric training journey, make stretching and mobility work a consistent part of your recovery program. With dedication and patience, you'll notice improvements in your flexibility, movement quality, and overall well-being, setting the stage for long-term success and enjoyment in your fitness pursuits.

# Rest and Sleep

Stress management is a crucial aspect of optimizing recovery and promoting overall well-being in the context of isometric training and beyond. Chronic stress can have a profound impact on both physical and mental health, impairing recovery, compromising performance, and increasing the risk of burnout and injury. By implementing effective stress management techniques, you can support optimal recovery, enhance your ability to adapt to the demands of isometric training, and improve your overall quality of life. Let's take an in-depth look at the importance of stress management and explore practical strategies for incorporating it into your recovery routine.

## 1. The Impact of Stress on Recovery and Performance

Stress is a natural response to the demands of life, but chronic or excessive stress can have negative consequences for recovery and performance:

a. Hormonal imbalances: Chronic stress can lead to elevated levels of cortisol, the primary stress hormone, which can interfere with muscle recovery, impair immune function, and disrupt sleep patterns.

b. Impaired recovery: High levels of stress can compromise the body's ability to repair and rebuild muscle tissue after exercise, leading to prolonged soreness, increased risk of injury, and impaired adaptations to training.

c. Decreased performance: Stress can negatively impact mental focus, motivation, and energy levels, leading to decreased performance during isometric training sessions and other activities.

d. Increased risk of burnout: Chronic stress can contribute to feelings of exhaustion, apathy, and decreased enjoyment of training and other activities, increasing the risk of burnout and abandonment of fitness goals.

## 2. Identifying Sources of Stress

To effectively manage stress, it is important to identify the sources of stress in your life:

a. Training-related stress: High-intensity isometric training, overtraining, and insufficient recovery can all contribute to training-related stress.

b. Work-related stress: Job demands, deadlines, and workplace conflicts can be significant sources of stress for many individuals.

c. Personal stress: Relationship difficulties, financial concerns, and health issues can all contribute to personal stress.

d. Environmental stress: Noise pollution, traffic, and other environmental factors can also contribute to overall stress levels.

## 3. Practical Stress Management Techniques

There are many effective techniques for managing stress and promoting relaxation and recovery:

a. Deep breathing: Practicing deep, diaphragmatic breathing can help activate the body's relaxation response and reduce feelings of stress and tension. Try taking slow, deep breaths for 5-10 minutes each day, focusing on the sensation of the breath moving in and out of the body.

b. Progressive muscle relaxation: This technique involves systematically tensing and relaxing different muscle groups in the body to promote feelings of relaxation and reduce muscle tension. Start at the toes and work your way up to the head, holding each tension for 5-10 seconds before releasing.

c. Meditation: Regular meditation practice can help calm the mind, reduce stress and anxiety, and promote feelings of well-being. Start with just a few minutes of meditation each day, focusing on the breath or a specific mantra, and gradually increase the duration over time.

d. Journaling: Writing down your thoughts and feelings can be a powerful tool for processing stress and promoting mental clarity. Try setting aside a few minutes each day to write about your experiences, challenges, and successes.

e. Time management: Effective time management can help reduce stress by ensuring that you have adequate time for both training and recovery, as well as other important activities and responsibilities

Try using a planner or scheduling app to prioritize tasks and allocate time efficiently.

## 4. The Importance of Sleep for Stress Management

Sleep is a critical component of stress management and overall recovery:

a. Restorative sleep: During sleep, the body releases hormones that promote muscle repair, tissue regeneration, and overall recovery. Adequate sleep is essential for optimizing the benefits of isometric training and reducing the risk of injury.

b. Stress reduction: Sleep helps reduce levels of cortisol and other stress hormones, promoting feelings of relaxation and well-being.

c. Cognitive function: Adequate sleep is essential for optimal cognitive function, including memory consolidation, learning, and decision-making. Impaired sleep can lead to decreased mental performance and increased stress levels.

To optimize sleep for stress management and recovery, aim for 7-9 hours of high-quality sleep each night. Establish a consistent sleep schedule, create a relaxing bedtime routine, and ensure that your sleep environment is dark, quiet, and comfortable.

## 5. Nutrition and Hydration for Stress Management

Proper nutrition and hydration can also play a role in stress management and overall recovery:

a. Balanced nutrition: Eating a balanced diet that includes plenty of fruits, vegetables, lean proteins, and healthy fats can help support optimal physical and mental function, reducing the impact of stress on the body.

b. Hydration: Adequate hydration is essential for overall health and can help reduce feelings of stress and fatigue. Aim for at least 8 glasses of water per day, and more during periods of intense training or heat exposure.

c. Caffeine and alcohol: While moderate consumption of caffeine can enhance mental alertness and performance, excessive intake can contribute to feelings of anxiety and stress. Similarly, while moderate alcohol consumption can have relaxation effects, excessive intake can impair sleep and recovery. Aim for moderation and be mindful of individual tolerance levels.

## 6. Seeking Professional Support

In some cases, stress management may require the support of a qualified professional:

a. Therapists and counselors: Mental health professionals can provide valuable support and guidance for managing stress, developing coping strategies, and addressing underlying mental health concerns.

b. Sports psychologists: For athletes and fitness enthusiasts, sports psychologists can help develop performance-enhancing mental skills, manage competition-related stress, and promote overall well-being.

c. Coaches and trainers: Qualified fitness professionals can provide guidance on optimizing training and recovery, managing training-related stress, and developing sustainable, long-term fitness habits.

Remember, seeking support is a sign of strength and self-awareness, not weakness. By taking a proactive approach to stress management and enlisting the support of qualified professionals when needed, you can optimize your recovery, enhance your performance, and promote overall well-being.

Incorporating stress management techniques into your recovery routine is essential for optimizing the benefits of isometric training and promoting overall physical and mental well-being. By identifying sources of stress, implementing practical management techniques, prioritizing sleep and nutrition, and seeking professional support when needed, you can reduce the negative impact of stress on your training and life.

Remember, stress management is a highly individualized process, and what works for one person may not work for another. Be patient, experiment with different techniques, and find what works best for you. With consistent practice and a commitment to self-care, you can develop resilience, enhance your recovery, and achieve your full potential in isometric training and beyond.

## Measuring Your Isometric Exercise Progress

Measuring your progress is a crucial component of any successful isometric exercise routine. By regularly assessing your performance and tracking your improvements over time, you can stay motivated, make informed adjustments to your training plan, and celebrate your achievements along the way. In this section, we'll take an in-depth look at the various methods for measuring your isometric exercise progress and provide practical strategies for incorporating these methods into your routine.

### 1. The Importance of Measuring Progress

Measuring your isometric exercise progress offers numerous benefits:

a. Motivation: Seeing tangible improvements in your performance can be a powerful motivator, helping you stay committed to your training routine and pushing through challenging plateaus.

b. Informed decision-making: By regularly assessing your progress, you can make data-driven decisions about your training plan, such as when to increase the difficulty of your exercises or when to incorporate new movements.

c. Identifying strengths and weaknesses: Tracking your progress can help you identify areas of strength and weakness in your isometric training, allowing you to focus your efforts on the areas that need the most improvement.

d. Celebrating achievements: Regularly measuring your progress provides opportunities to celebrate your successes and milestones, reinforcing the positive habits and behaviors that contribute to your overall fitness journey.

## 2. Methods for Measuring Isometric Exercise Progress

There are several effective methods for measuring your isometric exercise progress:

a. Maximum hold time: One of the most straightforward methods for measuring isometric exercise progress is to track your maximum hold time for each exercise. Aim to gradually increase your hold times over the course of your training program, setting specific time goals and celebrating when you achieve them.

b. Resistance levels: If you are using external resistance, such as resistance bands or weights, you can measure your progress by tracking the amount of resistance you are able to use for each exercise. Aim to gradually increase the resistance over time, while maintaining proper form and technique.

c. Perceived exertion: The Rating of Perceived Exertion (RPE) scale is a subjective measure of exercise intensity that can be used to track progress in isometric training.

The scale ranges from 6 (no exertion) to 20 (maximal exertion). Aim to maintain a consistent RPE throughout your training program, gradually increasing the difficulty of your exercises as your perceived exertion decreases.

d. Body measurements: While not a direct measure of isometric exercise performance, tracking changes in body measurements, such as waist circumference, can provide insight into the overall impact of your training program on your physical composition.

e. Performance tests: Regularly performing standardized performance tests, such as the plank hold test or the wall sit test, can provide an objective measure of your isometric exercise progress over time.

## 3. Tracking Your Progress
To effectively measure your isometric exercise progress, it's important to establish a consistent tracking system:

a. Training log: Keep a written or digital log of your isometric training sessions, including the exercises performed, hold times, resistance levels, and perceived exertion. Review your log regularly to identify trends and make informed adjustments to your training plan.

b. Progress photos: Take regular progress photos to visually document changes in your physical appearance and posture over time. Aim to take photos at consistent intervals, such as every 4-6 weeks, and in similar lighting and clothing conditions.

c. Measurement schedule: Establish a regular schedule for taking body measurements and performing performance tests, such as every 4-6 weeks. Consistency is key for accurately tracking changes over time.

d. Goal setting: Set specific, measurable goals for your isometric exercise progress, such as achieving a certain hold time for a particular exercise or increasing your resistance levels by a specific amount. Regularly review your goals and adjust them as needed based on your progress.

## 4. Interpreting Your Results

When measuring your isometric exercise progress, it's important to interpret your results in context:

a. Individual variability: Progress is highly individual and can be influenced by factors such as genetics, age, and training history. Don't compare your progress to others, but rather focus on your own improvements over time.

b. Non-linear progress: Progress in isometric training, like any form of exercise, is often non-linear. You may experience periods of rapid improvement followed by plateaus or even temporary declines in performance. This is a normal part of the training process and should not be a source of discouragement.

c. Consistency over perfection: Consistency in your training and tracking habits is more important than perfection. Even if you miss a training session or forget to log your progress, don't let it derail your overall efforts. Simply resume your routine and continue making forward progress.

## 5. Celebrating Your Achievements

Regularly celebrating your isometric exercise achievements is an important part of staying motivated and committed to your training routine:

a. Set milestones: Identify specific milestones in your isometric training journey, such as achieving a certain hold time or completing a certain number of training sessions, and celebrate when you reach them.

b. Reward yourself: Develop a system of rewards for achieving your isometric exercise goals, such as treating yourself to a massage or a new piece of workout gear. Choose rewards that align with your values and support your overall health and well-being.

c. Share your success: Consider sharing your isometric exercise achievements with supportive friends, family members, or online communities. Receiving recognition and encouragement from others can be a powerful motivator and help you stay accountable to your goals.

d. Practice self-compassion: Remember to be kind and compassionate with yourself throughout your isometric training journey. Progress is rarely linear, and setbacks are a normal part of the process. Celebrate your efforts and commitment, not just your outcomes, and approach challenges with curiosity and self-compassion.

Measuring your isometric exercise progress is a vital component of a successful training routine. By regularly assessing your performance, tracking your improvements, and celebrating your achievements, you can stay motivated, make informed decisions about your training plan, and ultimately achieve your fitness goals.

Remember, progress is highly individual and often non-linear. Focus on your own journey, be consistent in your tracking habits, and approach challenges with patience and self-compassion. With dedication and a commitment to self-improvement, you can unlock your full potential and achieve remarkable progress in your isometric training journey.

Staying accountable and consistent is crucial for long-term success in your isometric exercise journey. By developing strategies to hold yourself accountable and maintain consistency in your training routine, you can overcome obstacles, push through plateaus, and ultimately achieve your fitness goals. In this section, we'll explore the importance of accountability and consistency and provide practical strategies for incorporating these principles into your isometric training routine.

### 1. The Importance of Accountability and Consistency

Accountability and consistency are two key factors that contribute to success in any fitness endeavor, including isometric exercise:

a. Accountability: Holding yourself accountable means taking responsibility for your actions and commitments related to your isometric training routine. When you are accountable, you are more likely to follow through on your planned workouts, even when motivation is low or obstacles arise.

b. Consistency: Consistency refers to the regular, ongoing practice of your isometric exercise routine. When you are consistent in your training, you provide your body with the repeated stimulus needed to adapt and improve over time. Consistency is key for making progress and achieving long-term results.

## 2. Strategies for Staying Accountable

There are several effective strategies for holding yourself accountable to your isometric exercise routine:

a. Set specific goals: Develop clear, specific goals for your isometric training, such as achieving a certain hold time or mastering a particular exercise. Write your goals down and refer to them regularly to stay focused and motivated.

b. Create a schedule: Establish a regular schedule for your isometric workouts, and treat your training sessions as non-negotiable appointments. Block off time in your calendar and communicate your schedule to family members or roommates to minimize conflicts and distractions.

c. Track your progress: Regularly track your isometric exercise progress using a training log, progress photos, or other measurement tools. Seeing tangible evidence of your improvements over time can be a powerful motivator and help you stay accountable to your goals.

d. Find an accountability partner: Consider partnering with a friend, family member, or fellow isometric exercise enthusiast to hold each other accountable. Share your goals, check in regularly, and provide support and encouragement when motivation is low.

e. Join a community: Participate in online forums, social media groups, or in-person communities dedicated to isometric exercise. Surrounding yourself with like-minded individuals can provide accountability, motivation, and a sense of shared purpose.

## 3. Strategies for Staying Consistent

In addition to accountability, there are several strategies for maintaining consistency in your isometric exercise routine:

a. Start small: If you are new to isometric exercise or struggling with consistency, start with small, manageable goals and gradually build up over time. Focus on establishing the habit of regular training, even if your workouts are brief or less intense than you ultimately desire.

b. Make it enjoyable: Choose isometric exercises that you enjoy and look forward to doing. Incorporate variety in your routine to prevent boredom and maintain interest over time.

c. Prioritize recovery: Adequate rest and recovery are essential for maintaining consistency in your isometric training. Prioritize sleep, nutrition, and stress management to ensure that your body is well-prepared for each training session.

d. Plan for obstacles: Anticipate potential obstacles to your consistency, such as travel, illness, or changes in work or family obligations. Develop contingency plans and backup strategies to maintain your training routine even when circumstances are challenging.

e. Celebrate your efforts: Recognize and celebrate your efforts to stay consistent, even when progress is slow or setbacks occur. Focus on the process of showing up and putting in the work, rather than solely on outcomes or achievements.

## 4. Overcoming Setbacks and Plateaus

Even with the best intentions and strategies, setbacks and plateaus are a normal part of any fitness journey. Here are some tips for navigating these challenges and maintaining accountability and consistency:

a. Reframe setbacks as learning opportunities: When setbacks occur, resist the temptation to become discouraged or give up. Instead, approach challenges with curiosity and a growth mindset, looking for opportunities to learn and adapt.

b. Adjust your plan: If you experience a plateau or find yourself struggling to make progress, consider adjusting your isometric training plan. This may involve increasing the difficulty of your exercises, incorporating new movements, or modifying your recovery strategies.

c. Seek support: Don't hesitate to reach out to your accountability partner, training community, or a qualified fitness professional for support and guidance when facing setbacks or plateaus. Sometimes an outside perspective can provide valuable insights and help you get back on track.

d. Practice self-compassion: Be kind and understanding with yourself when setbacks or inconsistencies occur. Recognize that progress is rarely linear and that everyone experiences challenges along the way. Focus on the big picture and the overall trajectory of your journey, rather than getting caught up in temporary setbacks.

## 5. The Benefits of Accountability and Consistency

By prioritizing accountability and consistency in your isometric exercise routine, you can experience numerous benefits:

a. Improved performance: Consistent training provides the repeated stimulus needed for your body to adapt and improve over time. By staying accountable and showing up regularly for your workouts, you can make steady progress and achieve your performance goals.

b. Enhanced motivation: When you are accountable and consistent in your training, you build momentum and establish a positive feedback loop. Each successful workout reinforces your commitment and motivation, making it easier to stay on track over time.

c. Greater self-efficacy: Consistently following through on your commitments to your isometric exercise routine can boost your self-efficacy, or belief in your ability to succeed. This increased confidence can spill over into other areas of your life, such as work or personal relationships.

d. Long-term success: Accountability and consistency are essential for achieving long-term success in your isometric exercise journey. By making these principles a priority, you can transform temporary motivation into lasting habits and enjoy the benefits of a strong, healthy body for years to come.

Staying accountable and consistent is vital for unlocking your full potential and achieving your goals in isometric exercise. By setting specific goals, creating a schedule, tracking your progress, and utilizing other accountability and consistency strategies, you can overcome obstacles and make steady progress over time.

Remember, setbacks and plateaus are a normal part of the journey. Approach challenges with a growth mindset, seek support when needed, and practice self-compassion along the way. With dedication and a commitment to accountability and consistency, you can transform your isometric exercise routine into a powerful tool for personal growth and self-improvement.

Staying accountable and consistent is crucial for long-term success in your isometric exercise journey. By developing strategies to hold yourself accountable and maintain consistency in your training routine, you can overcome obstacles, push through plateaus, and ultimately achieve your fitness goals. In this section, we'll explore the importance of accountability and consistency and provide practical strategies for incorporating these principles into your isometric training routine.

## 1. The Importance of Accountability and Consistency

Accountability and consistency are two key factors that contribute to success in any fitness endeavor, including isometric exercise:

a. Accountability: Holding yourself accountable means taking responsibility for your actions and commitments related to your isometric training routine. When you are accountable, you are more likely to follow through on your planned workouts, even when motivation is low or obstacles arise.

b. Consistency: Consistency refers to the regular, ongoing practice of your isometric exercise routine. When you are consistent in your training, you provide your body with the repeated stimulus needed to adapt and improve over time. Consistency is key for making progress and achieving long-term results.

## 2. Strategies for Staying Accountable

There are several effective strategies for holding yourself accountable to your isometric exercise routine:

a. Set specific goals: Develop clear, specific goals for your isometric training, such as achieving a certain hold time or mastering a particular exercise. Write your goals down and refer to them regularly to stay focused and motivated.

b. Create a schedule: Establish a regular schedule for your isometric workouts, and treat your training sessions as non-negotiable appointments. Block off time in your calendar and communicate your schedule to family members or roommates to minimize conflicts and distractions.

c. Track your progress: Regularly track your isometric exercise progress using a training log, progress photos, or other measurement tools. Seeing tangible evidence of your improvements over time can be a powerful motivator and help you stay accountable to your goals.

d. Find an accountability partner: Consider partnering with a friend, family member, or fellow isometric exercise enthusiast to hold each other accountable. Share your goals, check in regularly, and provide support and encouragement when motivation is low.

e. Join a community: Participate in online forums, social media groups, or in-person communities dedicated to isometric exercise. Surrounding yourself with like-minded individuals can provide accountability, motivation, and a sense of shared purpose.

## 3. Strategies for Staying Consistent

In addition to accountability, there are several strategies for maintaining consistency in your isometric exercise routine:

a. Start small: If you are new to isometric exercise or struggling with consistency, start with small, manageable goals and gradually build up over time. Focus on establishing the habit of regular training, even if your workouts are brief or less intense than you ultimately desire.

b. Make it enjoyable: Choose isometric exercises that you enjoy and look forward to doing. Incorporate variety in your routine to prevent boredom and maintain interest over time.

c. Prioritize recovery: Adequate rest and recovery are essential for maintaining consistency in your isometric training. Prioritize sleep, nutrition, and stress management to ensure that your body is well-prepared for each training session.

d. Plan for obstacles: Anticipate potential obstacles to your consistency, such as travel, illness, or changes in work or family obligations. Develop contingency plans and backup strategies to maintain your training routine even when circumstances are challenging.

e. Celebrate your efforts: Recognize and celebrate your efforts to stay consistent, even when progress is slow or setbacks occur. Focus on the process of showing up and putting in the work, rather than solely on outcomes or achievements.

## 4. Overcoming Setbacks and Plateaus

Even with the best intentions and strategies, setbacks and plateaus are a normal part of any fitness journey. Here are some tips for navigating these challenges and maintaining accountability and consistency:

a. Reframe setbacks as learning opportunities: When setbacks occur, resist the temptation to become discouraged or give up. Instead, approach challenges with curiosity and a growth mindset, looking for opportunities to learn and adapt.

b. Adjust your plan: If you experience a plateau or find yourself struggling to make progress, consider adjusting your isometric training plan. This may involve increasing the difficulty of your exercises, incorporating new movements, or modifying your recovery strategies.

c. Seek support: Don't hesitate to reach out to your accountability partner, training community, or a qualified fitness professional for support and guidance when facing setbacks or plateaus. Sometimes an outside perspective can provide valuable insights and help you get back on track.

d. Practice self-compassion: Be kind and understanding with yourself when setbacks or inconsistencies occur. Recognize that progress is rarely linear and that everyone experiences challenges along the way. Focus on the big picture and the overall trajectory of your journey, rather than getting caught up in temporary setbacks.

## 5. The Benefits of Accountability and Consistency

By prioritizing accountability and consistency in your isometric exercise routine, you can experience numerous benefits:

a. Improved performance: Consistent training provides the repeated stimulus needed for your body to adapt and improve over time. By staying accountable and showing up regularly for your workouts, you can make steady progress and achieve your performance goals.

b. Enhanced motivation: When you are accountable and consistent in your training, you build momentum and establish a positive feedback loop. Each successful workout reinforces your commitment and motivation, making it easier to stay on track over time.

c. Greater self-efficacy: Consistently following through on your commitments to your isometric exercise routine can boost your self efficacy, or belief in your ability to succeed. This increased confidence can spill over into other areas of your life, such as work or personal relationships.

d. Long-term success: Accountability and consistency are essential for achieving long-term success in your isometric exercise journey. By making these principles a priority, you can transform temporary motivation into lasting habits and enjoy the benefits of a strong, healthy body for years to come.

Staying accountable and consistent is vital for unlocking your full potential and achieving your goals in isometric exercise. By setting specific goals, creating a schedule, tracking your progress, and utilizing other accountability and consistency strategies, you can overcome obstacles and make steady progress over time.

Remember, setbacks and plateaus are a normal part of the journey. Approach challenges with a growth mindset, seek support when needed, and practice self-compassion along the way. With dedication and a commitment to accountability and consistency, you can transform your isometric exercise routine into a powerful tool for personal growth and self-improvement.

Celebrating your achievements is an essential part of maintaining motivation, reinforcing positive habits, and fostering a sense of pride and accomplishment in your isometric exercise journey. When you take the time to acknowledge and celebrate your successes, both big and small, you create a positive feedback loop that can sustain your momentum and inspire continued progress. In this section, we'll explore the importance of celebrating your achievements and provide practical strategies for incorporating celebration into your isometric training routine.

## 1. The Importance of Celebrating Achievements

Celebrating your achievements offers numerous benefits for your physical, mental, and emotional well-being:

a. Reinforces positive habits: When you celebrate your successes, you reinforce the positive habits and behaviors that contributed to those successes. This reinforcement increases the likelihood that you will continue engaging in those habits, even when motivation is low or obstacles arise.

b. Boosts motivation and confidence: Celebrating your achievements can provide a powerful boost to your motivation and self-confidence. When you take the time to acknowledge your hard work and progress, you remind yourself of your capabilities and create a sense of pride and accomplishment that can fuel further efforts.

c. Provides perspective: In the midst of the day-to-day challenges and setbacks of isometric training, it can be easy to lose sight of the bigger picture. Celebrating your achievements helps provide perspective and reminds you of how far you have come, even when progress feels slow or difficult.

d. Enhances overall well-being: Celebrating your successes can contribute to a greater sense of overall well-being and life satisfaction. When you make a habit of acknowledging and savoring your achievements, you cultivate a more positive and appreciative mindset that can spill over into other areas of your life.

## 2. Strategies for Celebrating Achievements

There are many ways to celebrate your achievements in your isometric exercise journey. Here are some strategies to consider:

a. Set meaningful milestones: Identify specific, meaningful milestones in your isometric training routine and plan to celebrate when you reach them. These milestones could be related to performance (such as achieving a certain hold time), consistency (such as completing a certain number of workouts), or personal growth (such as overcoming a fear or plateau).

b. Create a rewards system: Develop a system of rewards for achieving your isometric training goals. These rewards could be tangible (such as a new piece of workout gear or a massage) or experiential (such as a day trip or a special outing with friends).

Choose rewards that align with your values and support your overall health and well-being.

c. Share your successes: Consider sharing your achievements with supportive friends, family members, or online communities. Receiving recognition and encouragement from others can be a powerful motivator and help you feel more connected and accountable in your journey.

d. Practice self-praise: Make a habit of praising yourself for your efforts and achievements, even when no one else is around. Use positive self-talk and affirmations to acknowledge your hard work and progress, and cultivate a sense of pride and self-appreciation.

e. Document your journey: Consider keeping a training journal or progress log to document your isometric exercise journey. Record your workouts, reflections, and achievements, and take time to review your entries periodically. Seeing tangible evidence of your progress can be a powerful motivator and reminder of your capabilities.

## 3. Celebrating vs. Boasting

While celebrating your achievements is important, it's equally important to distinguish between healthy celebration and unhealthy boasting or self-aggrandizement. Here are some tips for keeping your celebrations positive and productive:

a. Focus on the process: When celebrating your achievements, focus on the process of consistent effort and dedication that led to those successes, rather than solely on the outcomes themselves. Celebrate your commitment to your goals and your willingness to show up and do the work, even when it's challenging.

b. Maintain perspective: While it's important to acknowledge and celebrate your achievements, try to maintain a healthy perspective and avoid overstating or exaggerating your successes. Remember that progress is often non-linear and that setbacks and challenges are a normal part of any journey.

c. Celebrate others: In addition to celebrating your own achievements, make a habit of celebrating the successes and milestones of others in your community. Offering genuine support and encouragement to others can foster a sense of connection and positivity that benefits everyone.

d. Practice humility: When sharing your achievements with others, practice humility and avoid comparing yourself or competing with others. Remember that everyone's journey is unique and that success looks different for different people.

**4. Celebrating Effort and Progress, Not Just Outcomes**
One of the keys to effective celebration is to focus on effort and progress, not just outcomes or achievements. Here are some ways to celebrate the process of your isometric exercise journey:

a. Acknowledge your consistency: Celebrate your commitment to showing up and putting in the work, even on days when you don't feel motivated or energized. Consistency is a significant achievement in itself and deserves recognition.

b. Celebrate small wins: Look for opportunities to celebrate small wins and milestones along the way, such as mastering a new exercise, increasing your hold time by a few seconds, or completing a particularly challenging workout. These small victories add up over time and contribute to your overall progress.

c. Reframe setbacks as learning opportunities: When setbacks or failures occur, reframe them as valuable learning opportunities and celebrate your willingness to take risks and push yourself out of your comfort zone. Embrace the growth and resilience that comes from navigating challenges and setbacks.

d. Practice gratitude: Make a habit of practicing gratitude for your body, your health, and the opportunity to engage in isometric exercise. Celebrate the gift of movement and the ability to pursue your goals, regardless of your current level of fitness or achievement.

**5. The Ripple Effect of Celebration**
Celebrating your achievements in your isometric exercise journey can have a powerful ripple effect that extends beyond your training routine. Here are some ways that celebration can positively impact other areas of your life:

a. Improved self-esteem: Regularly celebrating your achievements can boost your self-esteem and self-confidence, which can translate to greater assertiveness, resilience, and success in other areas of your life, such as work or relationships.

b. Enhanced motivation in other pursuits: The positive feelings and increased self-efficacy that come from celebrating your isometric training successes can spill over into other areas of your life, providing motivation and inspiration to pursue your goals and dreams in other domains.

c. Strengthened relationships: Sharing your achievements with supportive friends and family members can strengthen your relationships and foster a sense of connection and shared purpose. Celebrating others' successes can also deepen your bonds and create a culture of positivity and encouragement.

d. Greater overall well-being: Celebrating your achievements and cultivating a positive, appreciative mindset can contribute to greater overall well-being and life satisfaction. When you make a habit of recognizing and savoring the good in your life, you create a foundation of joy and contentment that can weather any challenge.

Celebrating your achievements is a vital component of a successful and sustainable isometric exercise journey. By taking the time to acknowledge and celebrate your successes, both big and small, you reinforce positive habits, boost

# Conclusion

Congratulations on making it to the end of this comprehensive guide on isometric exercises! By now, you should have a deep understanding of the science, benefits, and practical applications of this powerful training method.

Throughout this book, we've explored the many ways that isometric exercises can transform your body, mind, and overall well-being. From building strength and muscle to enhancing endurance and joint stability, the benefits of isometric training are vast and far-reaching.

But perhaps even more important than the physical benefits are the mental and emotional rewards of embracing this journey. Isometric exercises teach us discipline, resilience, and the power of consistency. They challenge us to push beyond our perceived limits and discover new depths of inner strength and determination.

As you embark on your own isometric training journey, remember that progress is not always linear. There will be setbacks, plateaus, and moments of doubt. But with the right mindset and strategies, you have the power to overcome any obstacle and achieve your goals.

So stay committed to your journey, even when the path gets tough. Celebrate your achievements, both big and small, and use them as fuel for further growth and progress. Surround yourself with supportive individuals who believe in your potential and inspire you to be your best self.

Most importantly, remember that the ultimate goal of isometric exercise is not just to build a stronger body, but to cultivate a stronger, more resilient spirit. Embrace the challenges and lessons of this journey, and allow them to transform you from the inside out.

As you continue to integrate isometric exercises into your lifestyle, know that you are part of a growing community of individuals who are passionate about unlocking their full potential and living their best lives. Together, we can support and inspire each other to new heights of health, happiness, and success.

So go forth with confidence, armed with the knowledge, tools, and strategies you need to succeed. Embrace the power of isometric exercises, and watch as your body, mind, and spirit transform in ways you never thought possible.

Remember, your potential is limitless. Your strength is infinite. Your journey is just beginning.

Thank you for joining me on this incredible adventure. I can't wait to see where your isometric exercise journey takes you next.

To your health, happiness, and unstoppable success.